An Atlas of Investigation and Diagnosis
DEMENTIA

An Atlas of Investigation and Diagnosis

DEMENTIA

Daniel W McKeel, Jr
Alzheimer's Disease Research Center
Washington University School of Medicine
St Louis, Missouri, USA

Jeffrey M Burns
Alzheimer and Memory Program
University of Kansas School of Medicine
Kansas City, Kansas, USA

Thomas M Meuser
Alzheimer's Disease Research Center
Washington University School of Medicine
St Louis, Missouri, USA

John C Morris
Alzheimer's Disease Research Center
Washington University School of Medicine
St Louis, Missouri, USA

CLINICAL PUBLISHING

OXFORD

Clinical Publishing
an imprint of Atlas Medical Publishing Ltd
Oxford Centre for Innovation
Mill Street, Oxford OX2 0JX, UK

Tel: +44 1865 811116
Fax: +44 1865 251550
Email: info@clinicalpublishing.co.uk
Web: www.clinicalpublishing.co.uk

Distributed in USA and Canada by:
Clinical Publishing
30 Amberwood Parkway
Ashland OH 44805 USA

tel: 800-247-6553 (toll free within U.S. and Canada)
fax: 419-281-6883
email: order@bookmasters.com

Distributed in UK and Rest of World by:
Marston Book Services Ltd
PO Box 269
Abingdon
Oxon OX14 4YN UK

tel: +44 1235 465500
fax: +44 1235 465555
e mail: trade.orders@marston.co.uk

A catalogue record of this book is available from the British Library

ISBN-13 978 1 904392 37 8
ISBN-10 1 904392 37 7

The publisher makes no representation, express or implied, that the dosages in this book are correct. Readers must therefore always check the product information and clinical procedures with the most up-to-date published product information and data sheets provided by the manufacturers and the most recent codes of conduct and safety regulations. The authors and the publisher do not accept any liability for any errors in the text or for the misuse or misapplication of material in this work.

Printed by T G Hostench SA, Barcelona, Spain

Contents

Preface

Knowledge about the clinical, neuropsychological, neuro-imaging, biochemical, molecular, and neuropathological characterization of neurodegenerative dementing disorders is rapidly growing. This atlas was conceived as a compendium of clinical and neuropathological descriptions of these features and is intended to inform all who are interested in the dementing disorders, including students, postdoctoral trainees, health care professionals, practicing physicians, and scientists. The emphasis is on clinical and pathological differential diagnosis.

This atlas is not meant to be a comprehensive treatise but rather a focused review that can be used to gain a rapid and up-to-date perspective on key features of dementing neuro-degenerative disorders. The neuroimaging and pathologic illustrations and the literature citations in each chapter are selected to enhance the reader's understanding of disease expression and differential diagnostic features. We include both seminal and recent references with preference being given to reviews. We believe in establishing reliable clinico-pathological relationships that assist in arriving at an accurate final diagnosis as a critical element in the effort to assess new treatments and in presenting new research findings.

Each chapter includes summary tables of core clinical and neuropathologic features of the disease or disease family being discussed. An exhaustive coverage of each topic is beyond the scope of this monograph; several excellent books cover specific topics in more depth.

The atlas was authored by clinician-scientists from the Alzheimer's Disease Research Center (ADRC) at Washington University in St Louis, Missouri, and at the University of Kansas School of Medicine, in Kansas City, Kansas, USA. As such, it reflects the contributions of our many colleagues and collaborators who have influenced us in numerous important ways. Chief among these influences is the ADRC's focus in the clinical distinction of early-stage dementia from nondemented aging by eliciting evidence of intraindividual cognitive decline from previously attained levels and on the validation of these distinctions through clinicopathological correlations.

Chapter 1 is a clinical overview of dementing disorders. The diagnosis of these disorders focuses on Alzheimer's disease (AD) because it is by far the most common cause of dementia in older adults. The growing role of neuroimaging in clinical settings and in research is also discussed.

Chapter 2 presents an approach to the behavioral assessment of AD dementia with neuropsychological tests.

Chapter 3 addresses autopsy and histopathological methods used in the ADRC's Neuropathology Core to diagnose various adult dementias in over 1,050 brains from longitudinally characterized research subjects. Routine histopathologic, special dye and silver stains, and immunohistochemical techniques as well as specialized autopsy techniques for brain, cerebrospinal fluid, and pituitary gland removal are presented and illustrated. Selected staining protocols used in the ADRC Neuropathology Core laboratory are presented in the Appendix.

Chapter 4 covers the spectrum of aging-associated neuropathologic findings that form the necessary baseline for assessing abnormalities caused by dementing disorders. Even today, our knowledge base of these important features of healthy or 'normal' brain aging are incompletely defined.

Chapter 5 focuses on the neuropathology of AD. Our research indicates that AD pathology may begin in the sixth decade of life or even earlier with focal deposition of preamyloid and diffuse beta amyloid plaques, accompanied by very focal formation of pretangles and tangles in certain specific cerebral regions. The lesion profiles are associated with very mild, mild, moderate, and severe dementia as defined by the Clinical Dementia Rating (CDR), which was developed in 1982 by Leonard Berg, Charles Hughes, and colleagues at the predecessor to our ADRC and was updated by John C Morris in 1993. The chapter also discusses the roles of vascular disease and cerebral amyloid angiopathy and cerebrovascular lesions as they interact with other features of AD pathology.

The following chapters deal in turn with vascular dementia (Chapter 6), Lewy body dementias as synucleinopathies (Chapter 7), and frontotemporal dementia (FTD) syndromes as types of tauopathies (Chapter 8). Chapter 9 briefly surveys a number of less common dementing illnesses to provide readers with an idea of the full range of clinical conditions and pathologic lesions that are associated with dementia. It is our hope that readers will develop a sense of the interplay of clinical expressions of the various disorders with the underlying brain lesions that reflect disturbances of basic cellular and molecular processes.

We acknowledge with gratitude the large team of physicians in several specialties, nurses, psychologists, basic scientists, and others who make the ADRC a wonderfully stimulating environment in which to work and ultimately have made this book possible. We also are indebted to our research participants and their families who unstintingly give their time and support to the ADRC's efforts to conquer the dementing illnesses. The ADRC and its affiliated research programs have been supported for over two decades by the National Institute on Aging (Bethesda, Maryland), primarily through grants P01 AG03991 and P50 AG05681. Finally, we dedicate this atlas to our spouses, Louise, Jennifer, Christy, and Lucy, whose support makes our work possible.

Daniel W McKeel, Jr, MD
Jeffrey M Burns, MD
Thomas M Meuser, PhD
John C Morris, MD

Abbreviations

A4 amyloid beta peptide (synonyms a-beta, Aβ, BAP, 4 kd protein)

AAN American Academy of Neurology

AANP American Association of Neuro-pathologists

ACA anterior cerebral artery

ACTH adrenocorticotropic hormone

AD Alzheimer's disease

ADL activities of daily living

ADRC Alzheimer's Disease Research Center

ADRDA Alzheimer's Disease and Related Disorders Association

AGD argyrophilic grain disease

AHC anterior horn spinal cord

AIDS aquired immunodeficiency syndrome

ALS amyotrophic lateral sclerosis

AON anterior olfactory nucleus

apoE apolipoprotein E

AP anterior pituitary

APP amyloid precursor protein

AS atherosclerosis

aSYN alpha-synuclein

BCRS Brief Cognitive Rating Scale

BN ballooned neuron

BSE bovine spongiform encephalopathy

CA corpora amylacea

CAA cerebral amyloid (a-beta) angiopathy

CADASIL cerebral autosomal dominant arteriopathy with subcortical infarcts and leukoencephalopathy

CARASIL cerebral autosomal recessive arteriopathy with stroke and ischemic leukoencephalopathy

CBD corticobasal ganglionic degeneration

CC corpus callosum

CDI conformation-dependent immunoassay

CDR Clinical Dementia Rating

CERAD Consortium to Establish a Registry for Alzheimer's Disease

Chr. chromosome

CHS Cardiovascular Health Study

CJD Creutzfeldt-Jakob disease

CLB cortical Lewy body

CNS central nervous system

COW Circle of Willis

CP choroid plexus

CR Congo red

(pm)CSF (postmortem) cerebrospinal fluid

CT computed tomography

DAB diaminobenzidine (stain)

DAT dementia of Alzheimer's type

DBL double barrel lumen

DF dentate fascia

DG Dentate gyrus

DH2O distilled water

DIC differential interference contrast

DLB dementia with Lewy bodies

DLDH dementia lacking distinctive histopathology

DMN dorsal motor nucleus of the vagus nerve (X)

DN dystrophic neurite

DR dorsal raphe

DS Down's syndrome

DSM Diagnostic and Statistical Manual

DSP diffuse senile plaque

EEG electroencephalogram

EM electron microscopy

ERC-II entorhinal cortex layer II stellate cells

FFI fatal familial insomnia

FFPE formalin-fixed paraffin-embedded

fMRI functional magnetic resonance imaging

FTD frontotemporal dementia

FTDP-17 frontotemporal degeneration with parkinsonism linked to chromosome 17

fvFTD frontal variant frontotemporal dementia

GCI glial cell inclusions

GDS Global Deterioration Scale

GFAP glial fibrillary acidic protein

GM gray matter

GP-COG General Practitioner Assessment of Cognition

GSS Gerstmann–Scheinker–Sträussler disease

GVD granulovacuolar degeneration

HD Huntington's disease

HDDD hereditary dysphasic dementia with disinhibition

H&E hematoxylin eosin (stain)

HIPAA Health Insurance Portability and Accountability Act

HIV human immunodeficiency virus

HS hippocampal sclerosis

H-S Hallervorden–Spatz disease

ICA internal carotid artery

ICH intracerebral and cerebellar hemorrhage

IHC immunohistochemistry

IPD idiopathic Parkinson's disease

IQCODE Informant Questionnaire on Cognitive Decline in the Elderly

IRB Institutional Review Board

IVC intraventricular hemorrhage

LB Lewy body

LC locus ceruleus

LCN laminar cortical necrosis

LFB luxol fast blue

LN Lewy neurite

LP lumbar puncture

mab monoclonal antibody

MCA middle cerebral artery

MCI mild cognitive impairment

MID multi-infarct dementia

MMSE Mini-mental State Examination

MND motor neuron disease

MNI motor neuron disease-type inclusions

MRI magnetic resonance imaging

mRNA messenger ribonucleic acid

MS multiple sclerosis

MSA multiple system atrophy

NACC National Alzheimer Coordinating Center, Seattle, WA, USA

NBF neutral buffered formalin

NBIA-I neurodegeneration with brain iron deposition, type 1

NBM nucleus basalis of Meynert

NCL neuronal ceroid lipofuscinosis

NFP neurofibrillary pathology

NFT neurofibrillary tangle

NFTD neurofibrillary tangle dementia

NIA National Institute on Aging

NINCDS-ADRDA National Institute of Neurologic and Communicative Disorders and Stroke and the Alzheimer's Disease and Related Disorders Association

NNSP non-neuritic senile plaque

NPH normal pressure hydrocephalus

NSP neuritic senile plaque

NT neuropil thread

OPCA olivopontocerebellar ataxia

PAS periodic acid-Schiff

PCA posterior cerebral artery

PD Parkinson's disease

PDD Parkinson's disease dementia

PET positron emission tomography

PHF paired helical filaments

PHF tau hyperphosphorylated tau

PIB Pittsburgh compound-B

PiD Pick's disease

PMI postmortem interval

PML progressive multifocal leukoencephalopathy

PNFA progressive nonfluent aphasia

PNFD progressive nonfluent dysphasia

PP perforant pathway

PS1(2) presenilin 1(2)

PSFF paraffin sections of formalin fixed

PSP progressive supranuclear palsy

RBC red blood cell

REM rapid eye movement

RS Richardson's syndrome

RT real-time polymerase chain reaction

SAH subarachnoid hemorrhage

SBT Short Blessed Test

sCJD sporadic Creutzfeldt–Jakob disease

SD semantic dementia

SDH subdural hemorrhage

SGL supragranular layer

sIPD spontaneous idiopathic Parkinson's disease

SLE systemic lupus erythematosus

SN substantia nigra

SOD superoxide dismutase

SND striatonigral dementia

SP senile plaque

SPECT single photon emission computed tomography

STG superior temporal gyrus

TIA transient ischemic attack

TPA tissue plasminogen activator

TSE transmissible spongiform encephalopathy

TSH thyroid stimulating hormone
TSP total senile plaques
TTP thrombotic thrombocytopenic purpura
VaD vascular dementia
vCJD variant Creutzfeldt–Jakob disease
VH visual hallucinations
VPD vascular parkinsonism

V-R Virchow–Robins (perivascular spaces)
VTA ventral tegmental area
WAIS Wechsler Adult Intelligence Scale
WM white matter
WMI white matter infarct
WML white matter lesion

Chapter 1

Cognitive aging and dementia: an overview

Introduction

In 1907 Alois Alzheimer first described the clinical and pathologic features of the disease that now bears his name. Professor Alzheimer was among the first to correlate higher order cognitive dysfunction with changes in brain structure. Since then, the science of neuropathology has played an important role in the nosology of dementia, as Professor Alzheimer predicted:

'It is clear that there exist many more mental diseases than our textbooks indicate. In many such cases, a further histological examination must be effected to determine the characteristics of each single case. We must reach the stage in which the vast well-known disease groups must be subdivided into many smaller groups, each with its own clinical and anatomical characteristics' (translation by Bick & Amaducci, 1989).

Our understanding of disorders of higher cognitive function has advanced considerably in the last century, largely as a result of clinicopathologic studies such as Professor Alzheimer's. While molecular genetics and DNA analysis are now contributing importantly to disease classification, clinical and pathologic classifications will remain essential to interpreting the relationship of genotype and phenotype (Morris, 2000).

Dementia

Dementia is a clinical syndrome of acquired cognitive impairment produced by brain dysfunction. Dementia represents a decline from a higher level of cognitive function such that accustomed activities are accomplished less well or relinquished altogether. The American Academy of Neurology recommends the routine use of the Diagnostic and Statistical Manual (DSM) criteria for diagnosing dementia, which has been shown to be a reliable indicator of the presence of dementia (*Table 1.1*).

Dementia is a common disorder in older adults, involving as many as 10% of those over the age of 65 years. Increased life expectancy in the US and other developed countries has fueled an unprecedented growth in the elderly population

---

Table 1.1 Definition of dementia: DSM IV

- Impairment in short- and long-term memory, associated with impairment in abstract thinking, impaired judgment, other disturbances of higher cortical function, or personality change
- The disturbance is severe enough to interfere significantly with work or usual social activities or relationships with others

(American Psychiatric Association, 1994)

that is leading to dramatic increases in the incidence of dementia. The prevalence of the most common cause of dementia, Alzheimer's disease (AD), doubles every 5 years after the age of 65 years, and reaches nearly 50% after age 85 years (Evans *et al.*, 1989) (**1.1**). Currently, there are an estimated 4.5 million people in the US with AD and 20 million worldwide (World Health Organization); the incidence of AD has been projected to nearly triple in the US over the next 50 years (Hebert *et al.*, 2001) (**1.2**). The annual treatment costs of AD in the US are estimated at $100 billion with the cost to government agencies rising rapidly: Medicare spending on AD will grow to $49.3 billion (a 54% increase over the costs in 2000), and Medicaid spending will grow to $33 billion (an 80% increase over costs in 2000) (Prigerson, 2003).

Brain aging and dementia

It is well accepted that advancing age is associated with cognitive changes. When compared directly with younger subjects, older subjects tend to process information at a slower rate, manipulate and store information (working memory) less efficiently, and have declines in free-recall of word lists. On the other hand, cognitive declines with age are not universal to all types of cognition. For instance, crystallized intelligence (such as measures of knowledge and vocabulary) is stable across the lifespan (Park *et al.*, 2001) (**1.3**). Additionally, the magnitude of the deficits observed with age generally are small and do not appear to impair overall function appreciably or the ability to carry out activities of daily living (Rubin *et al.*, 1993).

The aging brain is associated with structural changes in even the healthiest individuals that may underlie some of the cognitive changes that are observed with age. Normal aging is associated with a slow and steady loss of brain tissue beginning in early adulthood and continuing over the lifespan (**1.4**) (Jernigan *et al.*, 2001; Bartzokis *et al.*, 2003; Fotenos *et al.*, 2005). White matter myelination continues into the fourth decade (Hildebrand *et al.*, 1993; Bartzokis *et al.*, 2001) but declines thereafter, with the occurrence of

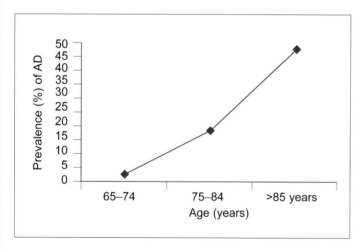

1.1 Prevalence of Alzheimer's disease in an aging population. Prevalence increases dramatically with age and approaches 50% of those over 85 years old. (Adapted from Evans *et al.*, 1989.)

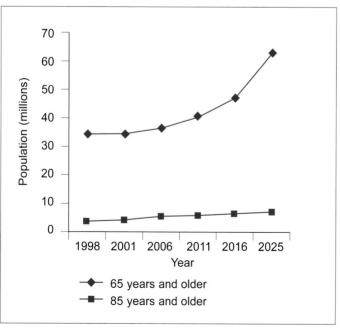

1.2 Population estimate for older adults in the US. The US Census Bureau (2000) projects the population of 65 years will increase dramatically by the year 2025 (middle series estimates). The 85 years and older group is the fastest growing segment of the population.

normal age-related breakdown in myelin (**1.5**) and the accumulation of changes in the white matter on magnetic resonance imaging (MRI) in older adults (**1.6**) (Longstreth *et al.*, 1996). Subclinical or 'silent' brain infarcts are present in up to 33% of nondemented older adults (Longstreth *et al.*, 1996; Vermeer *et al.*, 2002) and increase in prevalence with increasing age. These age-related brain changes are likely to play a role in the changes in cognition that occur

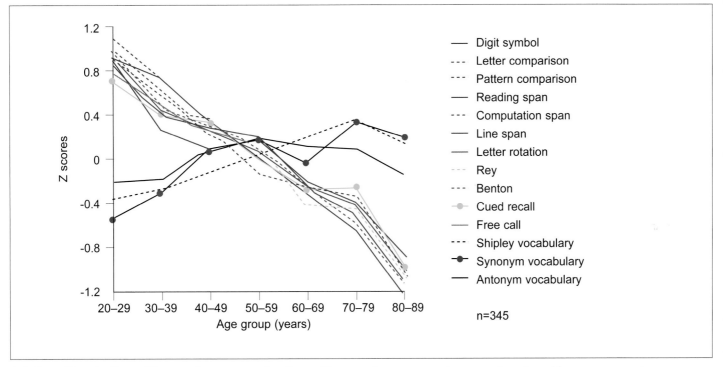

1.3 Cognitive decline with age. Some aspects of cognition, such as processing speed and working memory, are consistently reported to decline with age while others such as vocabulary, remain stable. Methodologic issues complicate these findings as longitudinal studies (following one individual over time) show less or no decline in cognition than cross-sectional studies (groups of individuals studied at one point in time). (Adapted from Park *et al.*, 2001.)

1.4 Cross-sectional plot of brain volume across the adult lifespan. Normal aging is associated in a slow and steady loss of brain tissue beginning in the seventh decade and extending over the lifespan. DAT: dementia of Alzheimer type; nWBV: normalized whole brain volume. (Adapted from Fotenos *et al.*, 2005.)

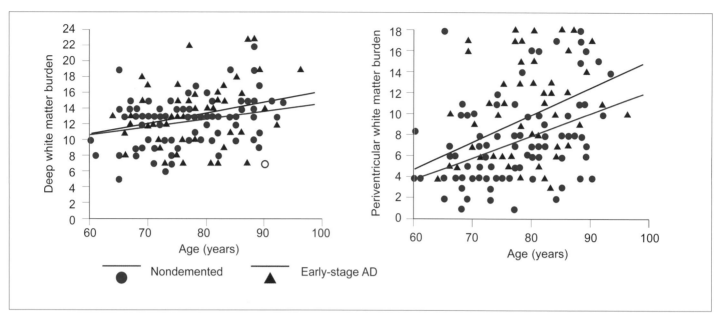

1.5 The burden of white matter lesions increases with age in individuals with early stage AD and healthy controls. (Adapted from Burns *et al.*, 2005.)

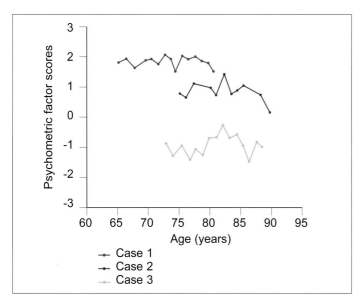

1.7 Stable cognitive performance with age in three nondemented controls. Factor score is an index of general cognitive performance generated from a battery of neuropsychologic tests. The large majority of a group of nondemented subjects followed for up to 15 years showed no decline in a standardized score of general cognitive performance.

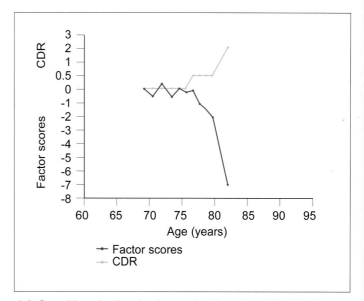

1.8 Cognitive decline in dementia. An abrupt decline in psychometric performance (green) occurs in this individual once subtle cognitive decline is detected (Clinical Dementia Rating (CDR) of 0.5, yellow). Stable cognitive performance is generally maintained up until the onset of a dementing illness, at which time a steep decline in performance occurs. Factor score is an index of cognitive performance. (Adapted from Rubin *et al.*, 1998.)

with advancing age. Additionally, there is a complex relationship between age-related brain changes and AD pathology. For instance, less AD neuropathology is required to produce clinically apparent dementia in the setting of cerebrovascular disease (Snowdon *et al.*, 1997; Esiri *et al.*, 1999; Zekry *et al.*, 2002). Thus, age-related brain changes are likely to contribute to the cognitive changes seen in healthy aging but also appear to influence the expression of AD in the aging population.

A central but unresolved issue is determining which cognitive changes can be accepted as part of normal aging. The mildest cognitive changes ascribed to early AD overlap considerably with cognitive performance in healthy aging

1.6 (Opposite.) Brain atrophy with age. Global atrophy is apparent in the brain of a 90-year-old nondemented man (**A**). The ventricles are significantly enlarged with prominent sulci. For comparison, a 39-year-old nondemented man (**B**) demonstrating smaller ventricles, fuller white matter, and less prominent sulci. (Courtesy of Randy L Buckner.)

individuals (Galasko *et al.*, 1990; Morris *et al.*, 1991; Devanand *et al.*, 1997; Herlitz *et al.*, 1997). This has, in part, prompted the consideration that aging and AD are part of the same spectrum (Ebly *et al.*, 1994), with cognitive decline and 'senility' suggested to be an inevitable result of the aging process. In fact, when strict criteria are employed to exclude even minimally demented individuals from longitudinal studies of cognitively normal elderly, psychometric performance is shown to be surprisingly stable (Howieson *et al.*, 1997; Rubin *et al.*, 1998; Storandt *et al.*, 2002). Thus, substantial cognitive decline need not be a part of truly healthy brain aging (Crystal *et al.*, 1988; Morris *et al.*, 1993; Howieson *et al.*, 1997; Rubin *et al.*, 1998; Haan *et al.*, 1999), suggesting that AD is not inevitable with age.

Clinical studies support a distinction between aging and AD. Cognitively healthy elderly individuals maintain generally stable cognitive performance when followed longitudinally over time (**1.7**). At dementia onset, however, a steep decline in cognitive performance occurs, suggesting the onset of disease is distinct from the aging process (**1.8**). While subtle changes can be expected with age, cognitive decline interfering even mildly with the ability to perform daily functions appears to be a marker of disease.

Alzheimer's disease and mild cognitive impairment

AD represents the most common cause of dementia, accounting for 55–70% of cases of dementia. AD is often accompanied by other age-related disorders. Vascular lesions and Parkinson's disease most commonly coexist with AD, each occurring in about 25% of AD cases. 'Pure' AD accounts for about 50–60% of clinically diagnosed cases of dementia. These concomitant disorders contribute to the expression of AD, as the histopathologic burden of AD lesions for a given level of dementia severity is lower when AD is mixed with other disorders (Nagy *et al.*, 1997; Snowdon *et al.*, 1997; Berg *et al.*, 1998). Given heterogeneity of clinical features and common pathologic overlap, the true occurrence of the non-AD dementias is difficult to ascertain. Dementia with Lewy bodies, vascular dementia, and the frontotemporal dementias are considered to be the most common forms of non-AD dementias (*Tables 1.2, 1.3*).

The term mild cognitive impairment (MCI) is one of many introduced to characterize the boundary of aging and dementia (Kral, 1962; Crook & Bartus, 1986; Flicker *et al.*, 1991; Levy, 1994; Graham *et al.*, 1997; Petersen *et al.*, 1999, 2001a). MCI was specifically intended to capture those patients destined to develop dementia (Flicker *et al.*, 1991). The onset of symptomatic AD is insidious and patients with AD almost always progress through a period of subtle cognitive impairments that do not interfere importantly with their daily functioning. Thus, the concept of MCI includes individuals in this prodromal stage that occurs prior to the diagnosis of overt dementia. Broadly defined, MCI includes (1) evidence of cognitive impairment; (2) preservation of general cognition and functional abilities; and (3) absence of diagnosed dementia. Prevalence estimates for MCI demonstrate considerable variability, ranging from 2.8% to as high as 23.4% (Ebly *et al.*, 1995; Ritchie *et al.*, 2001; Unverzagt *et al.*, 2001; Larrieu *et al.*, 2002; Lopez *et al.*, 2003). Estimates of the risk of 'conversion' from MCI to AD are also widely variable, ranging from 3.7% per year (Ritchie *et al.*, 2001) to 25% in selected samples (Flicker *et al.*, 1991; Dawe *et al.*, 1992). The wide variability in MCI prevalence and estimates of the risk for developing overt AD is due to differences in MCI definitions, study design (retrospective vs. prospective), and the sample studied (referral-based vs. population-based) (Luis *et al.*, 2003).

While MCI captures individuals with the earliest changes of AD or other forms of dementia (i.e. vascular dementia, frontotemporal dementia, dementia with Lewy bodies), it encompasses many different conditions including static cognitive impairment, the 'worried well', and reversible forms of cognitive dysfunction such as those related to depression or medical illnesses. In general, however, it seems clear that individuals with MCI progress to overt AD at a rate far above the baseline dementia incidence rate. Although the concept of MCI is not without controversy, it has served to focus attention on the delineation of the earliest symptoms of AD from the change of normal cognitive aging.

Table 1.2 Differential diagnosis of cognitive decline

- Neurodegenerative dementia (see *Table 1.3*)
- Cerebrovascular disorders:
  - Vascular dementia
  - Binswanger's disease
- Infectious disorders:
  - Chronic meningitis
  - Encephalitis:
    Human immunodeficiency virus
    Lyme disease
  - Progressive multifocal leukoencephalopathy
  - Neurosyphilis
  - Whipple's disease
- Toxic/metabolic encephalopathies
  - Drugs/medications
  - Endocrine: thyroid, parathyroid:
    Nutritional: B_{12} and thiamine deficiencies
    Fluid and electrolyte abnormalities
    Hypoglycemia
    Other: carbon monoxide, heavy metals (lead, mercury, arsenic, thallium)
- Inflammatory:
  - Vasculitis:
    Primary central nervous system vasculitis
    Systemic vasculitides:
      Systemic lupus erythematosus
      Polyarteritis nodosa
      Wegener's granulomatosus
      Churg–Strauss syndrome
      Sarcoidosis

- Demyelinating:
  - Multiple sclerosis
- Neoplastic:
  - Direct effects of primary and metastatic disease
  - Paraneoplastic syndromes
- Hydrocephalus
- Affective disorders (depression)
- Neurogenetic disorders:
  - Spinocerebellar ataxias
  - Dentatorubral-pallidoluysian atrophy
  - Hallervorden–Spatz disease
  - Gangliosidoses
  - Adult neuronal ceroid lipofuscinosis (Kuf's disease)
  - Mitochondrial encephalopathies
  - Porphyrias
  - Wilson's disease

Table 1.3 Neurodegenerative dementias

- Alzheimer's disease
- Dementia with Lewy bodies
- Vascular dementia
- Frontotemporal lobar degeneration:
  - Frontotemporal dementia
  - Semantic dementia
  - Progressive nonfluent aphasia
- Progressive supranuclear palsy

- Corticobasal degeneration
- Parkinson's disease with dementia
- Multiple system atrophy
- Huntington's disease
- Prion disorders:
  - Creutzfeldt–Jakob disease
  - Fatal familial insomnia
  - Gerstmann–Sträussler–Scheinker disease

Diagnosis and evaluation of dementing disorders

The key information for diagnosing dementia comes primarily from the clinical information, resting largely on determining whether cognitive decline is present to such a degree as to interfere with function in usual activities. The 2001 American Academy of Neurology (AAN) practice parameter on the diagnosis of dementia recommended the routine use of the DSM criteria (Knopman *et al.*, 2001b). The criteria's key principles include (1) cognitive decline; and (2) interference with functioning as the ultimate validation of the presence of dementia (*Table 1.4*). Assessing whether these criteria are met involves (1) evaluating the presenting problem; (2) obtaining information from someone who knows the patient well (i.e. obtaining an informant-based history); (3) physical and neurologic examinations; and (4) evaluation of the cognitive, behavioral, and functional status of the patient. Dementia remains a clinical diagnosis and no test replaces an assessment by an experienced physician.

Table 1.4 Clinical hallmarks of dementia

- Gradual onset
- Progressive decline
- Memory loss
- Other cognitive domains impaired
- Interferes with function

Table 1.5 Features suggestive of other dementing illness

- Parkinsonism → dementia with Lewy bodies, corticobasal degeneration
- Language:
    Naming impairment → progressive nonfluent aphasia
    Comprehension impairment → semantic dementia
- Apraxia → corticobasal degeneration
- Myoclonus → prion disease (Creutzfeldt–Jakob disease)

Importance of an informant-based history

Establishing a history of a significant cognitive decline must be individualized because each individual's usual activities vary according to native intelligence and their educational and occupational experiences. It is therefore important to gather information about cognitive changes from someone who knows the patient well, such as the spouse or a family member. The memory loss of early-stage AD is generally well compensated. Individuals may continue to perform independently in the community and symptoms may not be readily apparent in casual contact with others. Discussing cognitive changes with an attentive family member, relative, or friend is essential in making a confident diagnosis using their descriptions of cognitive changes to establish whether cognitive changes are interfering even mildly with the patient's usual function. The perceptions of a knowledgeable informant are sensitive and reliable for detecting early dementia (McGlone *et al.*, 1990; Koss *et al.*, 1993; Tierney *et al.*, 1996; Jorm, 1997; Carr *et al.*, 2000). Additionally, self-reported memory complaints do not correlate well with actual cognitive performance and are not a strong predictor of the development of dementia (Bolla *et al.*, 1991; Flicker *et al.*, 1993). On the other hand, these self-reported complaints should not necessarily be dismissed as benign as patients with early AD often retain some insight into their cognitive difficulties.

Neurologic examination

In mild and even moderate AD, focal neurologic abnormalities are infrequent and the neurologic examination is performed primarily to evaluate for any signs suggestive of another dementing illness (*Table 1.5*). The neurologic examination should therefore be focused on evaluating for the presence of focal upper motor neuron signs, extrapyramidal signs, and prominent aphasia and apraxia.

Mild impairments in language and praxis are commonly encountered in AD, although memory loss remains the prominent symptom. Language impairments often begin with mild word-finding difficulties, manifested as circumlocutions (substituting the desired word with a description or series of shorter words) and halting speech. Unexplained language impairments with relative sparing of memory may indicate the presence of a variant of frontotemporal lobar degeneration such as nonfluent progressive aphasia or semantic dementia.

Apraxia, a disorder of skilled movement despite intact strength, sensation, and coordination, will develop as typical AD progresses but is not a prominent early manifestation. Apraxia in mild AD patients is commonly characterized as substitution of the individual's hand as object, for instance using their fist to represent a hammer rather than grasping an imaginary hammer. Severe apraxia, often unilateral, may indicate corticobasal degeneration.

Focal neurologic deficits such as mild hemiparesis, unilateral visual field deficit, or Babinski sign may indicate the presence of significant vascular disease which commonly coexists with AD, and may play a role in the symptomatic expression of AD (Snowdon *et al.*, 1997). The presence of increased tone and a Parkinsonian gait early in the course may indicate dementia with Lewy bodies or Parkinson's dementia. Extrapyramidal signs are common in advanced AD but are generally not prominent early in the course; prominent unilateral extrapyramidal signs may indicate corticobasal degeneration. Prominent myoclonus may indicate Creutzfeldt–Jakob disease, especially if accompanying a rapidly progressive dementing illness, although myoclonus can also be encountered in the late stages of AD.

Laboratory and radiological evaluation

Structural neuroimaging is recommended in the form of either MRI or noncontrast computed tomography (CT). The basis of this recommendation is the evidence that up to 5% of patients with dementia have a clinically significant structural lesion that would not have been predicted based on the history or examination (Chui & Zhang, 1997). These potential lesions include brain neoplasms, subdural hematomas, or normal pressure hydrocephalus. However, fully reversible dementia due to unsuspected causes is rare. The AAN practice paramenter reported insufficient evidence to recommend single photon emission computed tomography (SPECT) or positron emission tomography (PET) in the routine evaluation of dementia patients. Additionally, PET and SPECT imaging have not been shown to be cost-effective for dementia diagnosis (McMahon *et al.*, 2000).

Depression, B_{12} deficiency, and hypothyroidism are common co-morbidities in patients with suspected

Table 1.6 Basic laboratory assessment for cognitive impairment

- Neuroimaging:
  - CT or MRI
- Laboratory:
  - Thyroid
  - Vitamin B_{12}
  - Syphilis (only if clinically indicated)

dementia, and screening for these treatable disorders is recommended (*Table 1.6*) (Knopman *et al.*, 2001). Depression coexists with AD in up to 12% of demented patients (Forsell and Winblad, 1998), and a few reports have attributed dementia to B_{12} deficiency and hypothyroidism (Clarfield, 1988). In most individuals, treatment of these disorders is unlikely to reverse cognitive deficits completely, and cognitive improvement in demented patients with B_{12} and thyroid replacement are equivocal (Knopman *et al.*, 2001a). Nevertheless, the high frequency of these co-morbidities and the potential for amelioration of cognitive symptoms necessitates screening. Routine screening for syphilis is no longer recommended, a change from the 1994 practice parameter (American Academy of Neurology/Quality Standards Subcommittee, 1994) unless syphilis risk factors or evidence of infection exists.

Psychometric/mental status testing

Mental status tests should be used primarily to confirm the presence of cognitive deficits and not as a method of diagnosis. Mental status tests cannot, certainly at the initial evaluation, indicate whether the individual has declined from previous levels of cognitive abilities nor determine the presence of impairment sufficient to interfere with accustomed activities. This information must be collected from the informant interview. Testing is useful in demonstrating a pattern of deficits consistent with an AD pattern (primary deficits in memory and executive function) and to monitor dementia progression over time through serial testing. Over-reliance on cognitive test performance in addition to failure to incorporate an informant's observations about an individual's cognitive function in relation to past abilities results in the under-recognition of mild AD.

The determination of normal and abnormal performance on psychometric tests uses arbitrary cutoff points and standard deviations for a group means of memory performance. These means are not always applicable to an individual. Cognitive tests, such as the Mini-mental State Examination (MMSE) (Folstein *et al.*, 1975) are influenced by age, education (Doraiswamy *et al.*, 1995), race (Manly *et al.*, 1998), and gender, and show large measurement error (*Table 1.7*). These factors often make cognitive tests insensitive to early-stage AD (Galasko *et al.*, 1990; Devanand *et al.*, 1997; Herlitz *et al.*, 1997). The performance of nondemented aging and very mild and mild AD individuals on widely used cognitive scales such as the MMSE and the Blessed Scale-cognitive portion (Blessed *et al.*, 1968) show considerable overlap between the groups. This suggests that over-reliance on neuropsychologic tests would exclude some individuals experiencing interference with their usual functions who are still performing within the arbitrary range of normal.

Summary

The key information for diagnosing dementia comes primarily from the clinical assessment. In establishing a diagnosis, clinicians should obtain a history from someone who knows the patient well as the perceptions of a knowledgeable informant are sensitive and reliable for detecting early dementia (McGlone *et al.*, 1990; Koss *et al.*, 1993; Tierney *et al.*, 1996; Jorm, 1997; Carr *et al.*, 2000). While brain aging is associated with structural and functional changes, cognitive changes seen normally with age are generally mild and should not be expected to interfere, even mildly, with an individual's accustomed activities of daily living.

There is currently a great interest in the potential utility of biomarkers, neuroimaging, and genetics in augmenting, or even replacing, the clinical diagnosis of dementing disorders. Clinical methods, however, remain the gold standard for the antemortem diagnosis of dementia and AD. Additionally, clinical and pathologic classifications will remain the backbone of interpreting these methods and in advancing our understanding of the complex interplay between genotype and phenotype.

Table 1.7 Selective cognitive instruments used in detection of dementia

Instrument (cutoff)	Sensitivity (%)	Specificity (%)
MMSE (<24) (Kukull *et al.*, 1994)	63	96
MMSE (bottom 10%) (Ganguli *et al.*, 1993)	49	92
MMSE (decline of 4 points)/1–4 years (Tangalos *et al.*, 1996)	82	99
Seven-minute screen (Solomon *et al.*, 1998)	92	96
Clock drawing test (Shulman, 2000)	85	85
CDR (Juva *et al.*, 1995)	92	94
IQCODE (Fuh *et al.*, 1995)	89	88

CDR: Clinical Dementia Rating Scale; IQCODE: Informant Questionnaire on Cognitive Decline in the Elderly.
(From Petersen *et al.*, 2001b)

References

American Academy of Neurology/Quality Standards Subcommittee (1994). Practice parameter for diagnosis and evaluation of dementia. *Neurology* **44**:2203–2206.

American Psychiatric Association (1994). *Diagnostic and Statistical Manual of Mental Disorders*. Washington, DC: American Psychiatric Association.

Bartzokis G, Beckson M, Lu PH, *et al.* (2001). Age-related changes in frontal and temporal lobe volumes in men: a magnetic resonance imaging study. *Arch. Gen. Psychiatry* **58**:461–465.

Bartzokis G, Cummings JL, Sultzer D, *et al.* (2003). White matter structural integrity in healthy aging adults and patients with Alzheimer disease: a magnetic resonance imaging study. *Arch. Neurol.* **60**:393–398.

Berg L, McKeel DW Jr., Miller JP, *et al.* (1998). Clinicopathologic studies in cognitively healthy aging and Alzheimer disease: relation of histological markers to dementia severity, age, sex, and apolipoprotein E genotype. *Arch. Neurol.* **55**:326–335.

Bick KL, Amaducci L (1989). *The Early Story of Alzheimer's Disease*. Liviana Press, Padova.

Blessed G, Tomlinson BE, Roth M (1968). The association between quantitative measures of dementia and of senile change in the cerebral grey matter of the elderly subjects. *Br. J. Psychiatry* **114**:797–811.

Bolla KI, Lindgren KN, Bonaccorsy C, *et al.* (1991). Memory complaints in older adults: fact or fiction? *Arch. Neurol.* **48**:61–64.

Burns JM, Church JA, Johnson DK, *et al.* (2005). White matter lesions are prevalent but differentially related with cognition in aging and early Alzheimer disease. *Arch Neurol* **62**(12):1870–1876.

Carr DB, Gray S, Baty J, *et al.* (2000). The value of informant vs. individual's complaints of memory impairment in early dementia. *Neurology* **55**:1724–1726.

Chui H, Zhang Q (1997). Evaluation of dementia: a systematic study of the usefulness of the American Academy of Neurology's practice parameters. *Neurology* **49**:925–935.

Clarfield AM (1988). The reversible dementias: do they reverse? *Ann. Intern. Med.* **109**:476–486.

Crook TH, Bartus RT (1986). Age-associated memory impairment: proposed diagnostic criteria and measures of clinical change; Report of a National Institute of Mental Health work group. *Dev. Neuropsychol.* **2**:261–276.

Crystal H, Dickson D, Fuld P, *et al.* (1988). Clinico-pathologic studies in dementia: nondemented subjects with pathologically confirmed Alzheimer's disease. *Neurology* **38**:1682–1687.

Dawe B, Procter A, Philpot M (1992). Concepts of mild memory impairment in the elderly and their relationship to dementia: a review. *Int. J. Geriatr. Psychiatry* **7**:473–479.

Devanand DP, Folz M, Gorlyn M, *et al.* (1997). Questionable dementia: clinical course and predictors of outcome. *J. Am. Geriatr. Soc.* **45**:321–328.

Doraiswamy PM, Krishen A, Stallone F, *et al.* (1995). Cognitive performance on the Alzheimer's disease assessment scale: effect of education. *Neurology* **45**:1980–1984.

Ebly EM, Hogan DB, Parhad IM (1995). Cognitive impairment in the nondemented elderly. Results from the Canadian Study of Health and Aging. *Arch. Neurol.* **52**:612–619.

Ebly EM, Parhad IM, Hogan DB, *et al.* (1994). Prevalence and types of dementia in the very old. Results from the Canadian Study of Health and Aging. *Neurology* **44**:1593–1600.

Esiri MM, Nagy Z, Smith MZ, *et al.* (1999). Cerebrovascular disease and threshold for dementia in the early stages of Alzheimer's disease. *Lancet* **354**:919–920.

Evans DA, Funkenstein HH, Albert MS, *et al.* (1989). Prevalence of Alzheimer's disease in a community population of older persons: higher than previously reported. *JAMA* **262**:2551–2556.

Flicker C, Ferris SH, Reisberg B (1991). Mild cognitive impairment in the elderly: predictors of dementia. *Neurology* **41**:1006–1009.

Flicker C, Ferris SH, Reisberg B (1993). A longitudinal study of cognitive function in elderly persons with subjective memory complaints. *J. Am. Geriatr. Soc.* **41**:1029–1032.

Folstein MF, Folstein SE, McHugh PR (1975). Mini-mental state: a practical method for grading the cognitive state of patients for the clinicians. *J. Psychiatr. Res.* **12**:189–198.

Forsell Y, Winblad B (1998). Major depression in a population of demented and nondemented older people: prevalence and correlates. *J. Am. Geriatr. Soc.* **46**:27–30.

Fotenos AF, Snyder AZ, Girton LE, *et al.* (2005). Normative estimates of cross-sectional and longitudinal brain volume decline in aging and AD. *Neurology* **64**:1032–1039.

Fuh JL, Teng EL, Lin KN, *et al.* (1995). The Informant Questionnaire on Cognitive Decline in the Elderly (IQCODE) as a screening tool for dementia for a predominantly illiterate Chinese population. *Neurology* **45**:92–96.

Galasko D, Klauber MR, Hofstetter R (1990). The Mini-mental state examination in the early diagnosis of Alzheimer's disease. *Arch. Neurol.* **47**:49–52.

Ganguli M, Belle S, Ratcliff G, *et al.* (1993). Sensitivity and specificity for dementia of population-based criteria for cognitive impairment: the MoVIES project. *J. Gerontol.* **48**:M152–M161.

Graham JE, Rockwood K, Beattie LB, *et al.* (1997). Prevalence and severity of cognitive impairment with and without dementia in an elderly population. *Lancet* **349**:1793–1796.

Haan MN, Shemanki L, Jagust WJ, *et al.* (1999). The role of APOE e4 in modulating effects of other risk factors for cognitive decline in elderly persons. *JAMA* **282**:40–46.

Hebert LE, Beckett LA, Scherr PA, *et al.* (2001). Annual incidence of Alzheimer disease in the United States projected to the years 2000 through 2050. *Alz. Dis. Assoc. Disord.* **15**:169–173.

Herlitz A, Small BJ, Fratiglioni L, *et al.* (1997). Detection of mild dementia in community surveys. *Arch. Neurol.* **54**:319–324.

Hildebrand C, Remahl S, Persson H, *et al.* (1993). Myelinated nerve fibres in the CNS. *Prog. Neurobiol.* **40**:319–384.

Howieson DB, Dame A, Camicioli R, *et al.* (1997). Cognitive markers preceding Alzheimer's dementia in the healthy oldest old. *J. Am. Geriatr. Soc.* **45**:584–589.

Jernigan TL, Archibald SL, Fennema-Notestine C, *et al.* (2001). Effects of age on tissues and regions of the cerebrum and cerebellum. *Neurobiology of Aging* **22**:581–594.

Jorm AF (1997). Methods of screening for dementia: a meta-analysis of studies comparing an informant questionnaire with a brief cognitive test. *Alz. Dis. Assoc. Disord.* **11**:158–162.

Juva K, Sulkava R, Erkinjuntti T, *et al.* (1995). Usefulness of the Clinical Dementia Rating scale in screening for dementia. *Int. Psychogeriatr.* **7**:17–24.

Knopman DS, DeKosky ST, Cummings JL, *et al.* (2001). Practice parameter: diagnosis of dementia (an evidence-based review). Report of the Quality Standards Subcommittee of the American Academy of Neurology. *Neurology* **56**:1143–1153.

Koss E, Patterson MB, Ownby R, *et al.* (1993). Memory evaluation in Alzheimer's disease: caregivers' appraisals and objective testing. *Arch. Neurol.* **50**:92–97.

Kral VA (1962). Senescent forgetfulness: benign and malignant. *Can. Med. Assoc. J.* **86**:257–260.

Kukull WA, Larson EB, Teri L, *et al.* (1994). The mini-mental state examination score and the clinical diagnosis of dementia. *J. Clin. Epidemiol.* **47**:1061–1067.

Larrieu S, Letenneur L, Orgogozo JM, *et al.* (2002). Incidence and outcome of mild cognitive impairment in a population-based prospective cohort. *Neurology* **59**:1594-1599.

Levy R (1994). Aging-associated cognitive decline. *Int. Psychogeriatr.* **6**:63-68.

Longstreth WT, Manolio TA, Arnold A, *et al.* (1996). Clinical correlates of white matter findings on cranial magnetic resonance imaging of 3301 elderly people: The Cardiovascular Health Study. *Stroke* **27**:1274–1282.

Lopez OL, Jagust WJ, Dulberg C, *et al.* (2003). Risk factors for mild cognitive impairment in the Cardiovascular Health Study Cognition Study: Part 2. *Arch. Neurol.* **60**:1394–1399.

Luis CA, Loewenstein DA, Acevedo A, *et al.* (2003). Mild cognitive impairment: directions for future research. *Neurology* **61**:438–444.

Manly JJ, Jacobs DM, Sano M, *et al.* (1998). Cognitive test performance among nondemented elderly African Americans and whites. *Neurology* **50**:1238–1245.

McGlone J, Gupta S, Humphrey D, *et al.* (1990). Screening for early dementia using memory complaints from patients and relatives. *Arch. Neurol.* **47**:1189–1193.

McMahon PM, Araki SS, Neumann PJ, *et al.* (2000). Cost-effectiveness of functional imaging tests in the diagnosis of Alzheimer disease. *Radiology* **217**:58–68.

Morris JC (2000). Nosology of dementia. In: *Neurologic Clinics*. ST DeKosky (ed). W.B. Saunders Company, Philadelphia, pp. 773–788.

Morris JC, Edland S, Clark C, *et al.* (1993). The Consortium to Establish a Registry for Alzheimer's Disease (CERAD). Part IV. Rates of cognitive change in the longitudinal assessment of probable Alzheimer's disease. *Neurology* **43**:2457–2465.

Morris JC, McKeel DW Jr., Storandt M, *et al.* (1991). Very mild Alzheimer's disease: informant-based clinical, psychometric, and pathological distinction from normal aging. *Neurology* **41**:469-478.

Nagy Z, Esiri MM, Jobst KA, *et al.* (1997). The effects of additional pathology on the cognitive deficit in Alzheimer disease. *J. Neuropathol. Exp. Neurol.* **56**:165–170.

Park DC, Plk TA, Mikels, *et al.* (2001). Cerebral aging: brain and behavioral models of cognitive function. *Dialog. Clin. Neurosci.* **3**:151–165.

Petersen RC, Smith GE, Waring SC *et al.* (1999). Mild cognitive impairment – clinical characterization and outcome. *Arch. Neurol.* **56**(3):303-3-8.

Petersen RC, Doody R, Kurz A, *et al.* (2001a) Current concepts in mild cognitive impairment. *Arch. Neurol.* **58**(12):1985–1992.

Petersen RC, Stevens JC, Ganguli M, *et al.* (2001b). Practice parameter: Early detection of dementia: mild cognitive impairment (an evidence-based review). Report of the Quality Standards Subcommittee of the American Academy of Neurology. *Neurology* **56**:1133–1142.

Prigerson HG (2003). Costs to society of family caregiving for patients with end-stage Alzheimer's disease. *N. Engl. J. Med.* **349**:1891–1892.

Ritchie K, Artero S, Touchon J (2001). Classification criteria for mild cognitive impairment. A population-based validation study. *Neurology* **56**:37–42.

Rubin EH, Storandt M, Miller JP, *et al.* (1993). Influence of age on clinical and psychometric assessment of subjects with very mild or mild dementia of the Alzheimer type. *Arch. Neurol.* **50**:380–383.

Rubin EH, Storandt M, Miller JP, *et al.* (1998). A prospective study of cognitive function and onset of dementia in cognitively healthy elders. *Arch. Neurol.* **55**:395–401.

Shulman K (2000). Clock-drawing: is it the ideal cognitive screening test? *Int. J. Geriatr. Psychiatry* **15**:548–561.

Snowdon DA, Greiner LH, Mortimer JA, *et al.* (1997). Brain infarction and the clinical expression of Alzheimer disease. *JAMA* **277**:813–817.

Solomon PR, Hirschoff A, Kelly B, *et al.* (1998) A 7 minute neurocognitive screening battery highly sensitive to Alzheimer's disease. *Arch. Neurol.* **55**:349–355.

Storandt M, Grant EA, Miller JP, *et al.* (2002). Rates of progression in mild cognitive impairment and early Alzheimer's disease. *Neurology* **59**:1034–1041.

Tangalos EG, Smith GE, Ivnik RJ, *et al.* (1996) The Mini-Mental State Examination in general medical practice: clinical utility and acceptance. *Mayo Clin. Proc.* **71**:829–837.

Tierney MC, Szalai JP, Snow WG, *et al.* (1996). The prediction of Alzheimer disease. *Arch. Neurol.* **53**:423–427.

Unverzagt FW, Gao S, Baiyewu O, *et al.* (2001). Prevalence of cognitive impairment: data from the Indianapolis Study of Health and Aging. *Neurology* **57**:1655–1662.

Vermeer SE, Koudstaal PJ, Oudkerk M, *et al.* (2002). Prevalence and risk factors of silent brain infarcts in the population-based Rotterdam Scan Study. *Stroke* **33**:21–25.

Zekry D, Duyckaerts C, Moulias R, *et al.* (2002). Degenerative and vascular lesions of the brain have synergistic effects in dementia of the elderly. *Acta Neuropathol. (Berl.)* **103**:481–487.

Chapter 2

Interviewing, screening, and staging of dementia: a focus on Alzheimer's disease

Introduction

'That January, my fifty-seventh birthday, was pleasant and eventful and I began to adjust to middle age ... I was active and happy ... Then came a beautiful spring day later that year. It was the day after the tests were finished and the results reviewed. It was the day that I was diagnosed with Alzheimer's. What time had now hidden was now revealed. Genetic secrets, locked inside before my birth, were now in the open. I became a new member in a parade of horror created by Alzheimer's' (DeBaggio, 2002, p. 1).

So begins a moving account of early-onset Alzheimer's disease (AD) by Thomas DeBaggio, a commercial herb grower and author from Virginia, US. For DeBaggio and millions like him in the US and across the globe, the advent of AD is a harsh reality. Minor problems with recent memory at first give way, over time, to generalized cognitive and functional decline, ending years later in profound loss of individual and interpersonal identity. Although affected individuals, like DeBaggio, may retain reasonable awareness of the disease and its impact early on, within months to a few years such awareness wanes, and the extended family is left to march in the 'parade of horror' alone. The affected individual is present in body, a subject of notice and care, but cognitively separate from the day-to-day realities of constant supervision, visits to the doctor, alterations in daily routine to accommodate new deficits, placement in a long-term care facility, and so on. AD is a disease of the individual *and* the family.

The early signs and symptoms of clinical AD are subtle and often difficult to distinguish from changes expected in normal aging, disturbances of mood, and/or quirks of personality. Close family members are typically the first to notice one or more warning signs (*Table 2.1*), but may not act to obtain a diagnosis until a number of these signs are evident and appreciated. Also, individuals with early AD will tend to compensate for deficits (e.g. by writing down information to be remembered, making more extensive use of a calendar), as well as downplaying or otherwise explaining away problems observed by others. Such efforts may further delay initiation of an evaluation process. In addition, local relatives may perceive a problem much earlier than those living at a distance. Disagreements can arise in a family network about what is going on and if medical intervention is truly needed. Despite such factors, the impetus for an older adult to be evaluated medically for memory loss and dementia typically rests with the family. When a family member raises a concern, the clinician providing care would do well to pay attention.

Once an evaluation is arranged and positive results known, family caregivers are forced, ready or not, to confront the harsh realities of AD: a prospect of progressive decline and a likelihood of increasing demands for care and support over time. The experience of family caregivers has been labeled 'the long goodbye' in a number of publications, most recently by President Ronald Reagan's daughter, Patti Davis (Davis, 2004). One of the most challenging aspects for family members is an ever-present and progressive loss of relationship with the affected individual. Vibrant, engaged loved ones gradually change into distant, superficial shells of their former selves. Close relatives, spouses, and adult children especially, have been shown to experience significant grief reactions in response to such losses (Meuser & Marwit, 2001; Marwit & Meuser, 2002). Providing care to a person with dementia is a stressful, burdensome

Table 2.1 Ten warning signs of AD

- *Memory loss:* one of the most common early signs of dementia is forgetting recently learned information. While it is normal to forget appointments, names, or telephone numbers, those with dementia will forget such things more often and not remember them later.
- *Difficulty performing familiar tasks:* people with dementia often find it hard to complete everyday tasks that are so familiar we usually do not think about how to do them. A person with AD may not know the steps for preparing a meal, using a household appliance, or participating in a lifelong hobby.
- *Problems with language:* everyone has trouble finding the right word sometimes, but a person with AD often forgets simple words or uses word substitutes, making his or her speech or writing hard to understand. If a person with AD is unable to find his or her toothbrush, for example, the individual may ask for 'that thing for my mouth'.
- *Disorientation to time and place:* it is normal to forget the day of the week or where you're going. People with AD can become lost on their own street. They may forget where they are and how they got there, and may not know how to get back home.
- *Poor or decreased judgement:* no one has perfect judgment all of the time. Those with AD may dress without regard to the weather, wearing several shirts on a warm day or very little clothing in cold weather. Those with dementia often show poor judgment about money, giving away large sums to telemarketers or paying for home repairs or products they don't need.

- *Problems with abstract thinking:* balancing a checkbook is a task that can be challenging for some. A person with AD may forget what the numbers represent and what needs to be done with them.
- *Misplacing things:* anyone can temporarily misplace a wallet or key. A person with AD may put things in unusual places, like an iron in the freezer or a wristwatch in the sugar bowl.
- *Changes in mood or behavior:* everyone can become sad or moody from time to time. Someone with AD can show rapid mood swings, from calm to tears to anger, for no apparent reason.
- *Changes in personality:* personalities ordinarily change somewhat with age. A person with AD can change dramatically, becoming extremely confused, suspicious, fearful, or dependent on a family member.
- *Loss of initiative:* it is normal to tire of housework, business activities, or social obligations at times. The person with AD may become very passive, sitting in front of the television for hours, sleeping more than usual, or not wanting to do usual activities.

(Adapted from Alzheimer's Association, 2004. Available on-line at http://www.alz.org/AboutAD/Warning.asp)

experience all around. Grief may be most acute and troublesome for adult children at the moderate stage when in-home care demands are high and huge personal adjustments are required, whereas spouse caregivers appear to experience a peak in grief following long-term care placement, often viewed as symbolic of failure ('I wasn't a good enough caregiver to keep my loved one at home') or of death itself ('My marriage is essentially over ... now where am I?'). In addition to grief and burden, caregivers also face an increased risk of physical health problems, disturbed sleep, anxiety, and depression (Connell *et al.*, 2001).

Role of the clinician

Physicians and other providers of medical care to older adults will, at one time or another, be involved in the recognition of key dementia symptoms, assessment towards a diagnosis, initiation and management of treatment, and provision of supportive, behavioral, and psychosocial care to patients and family members alike. The provision of such comprehensive services is not a simple matter and additional training is often helpful. Continuing education providers are increasingly offering dementia-specific educational opportunities (Meuser *et al.*, 2004). Community organizations (e.g. Alzheimer's Association: http://www.alz.org) and government-funded agencies (e.g. Area Agencies on Aging: http://www.n4a.org) are available to help by providing educational information, supportive services including support groups and respite programs, and referral assistance to patients and families.

In order to make a diagnosis of clinical AD, the clinician must show that significant impairment exists in memory functioning and in at least one other cognitive domain (e.g. language, orientation, executive functioning, visual-spatial skills). In addition, such deficits must be associated with decrements in daily life functioning (DSM-IV Criteria, American Psychiatric Association, 1994). In other words, to qualify for a diagnosis of AD, the patient must demonstrate both objective and subjective impairment, with deficits apparent on cognitive testing (and/or from history) and through observations of a family member or close associate.

The detection of cognitive functional deficits in dementia is not difficult *per se*, but does require an investment of time and a willingness to go beyond the typical brief office examination. Extra information is needed, both from the identified patient and an informant, typically a spouse, child, or other close family member. In the sections below, the evaluative and diagnostic approach, application of screening measures, staging of impairment level, and clinical dementia care as a function of patient and family needs are discussed.

Diagnosis of inclusion

It used to be the case that AD was considered a *diagnosis of exclusion* (Keefover, 1990). The clinician would test for, and otherwise rule out, alternative causes for observed symptoms. Tests of thyroid function, vitamin B_{12} level, hypertension, stroke, tumor, and so on, would be pursued first. If, after extensive testing, a metabolic or other acute cause could not be identified, it was assumed by process of elimination that AD was the likely cause of observed cognitive functional decline. The ultimate confirmation, however, would need to wait until histologic examination of brain tissue after death. A number of long-standing community brain banks, for example, continue to offer autopsy services to families for diagnostic confirmation and assessment of genetic risk (Murphy & Ravina, 2003).

Over the past 15–20 years, the diagnosis of AD has shifted to become a *diagnosis of inclusion* (Small *et al.*, 1997). Great strides have been made in identifying symptom and progression patterns. Accepted diagnostic criteria are readily available (e.g. Knopman *et al.*, 2001). It is now possible to diagnose uncomplicated or 'pure' cases of dementia of Alzheimer's type (DAT) with a high degree of accuracy, 85–90% in specialty centres (Morris, 2003). DAT accounts for as many as 65–70% of all cases of dementia among adults aged 65 years and older. Differential diagnosis of mixed dementia (i.e. when Alzheimer's disease co-exists with another neurodegenerative disease process) is more complicated, especially for nonspecialists, and accuracy rates are somewhat lower.

It is important to recognize that AD is a condition of aging. The risk of developing AD increases with advancing age, especially after age 70 years. The prevalence of AD under age 50 years, for example, is less than 2%. The typical cause of AD at this young age is familial transmission of a rare causal genetic mutation (Pastor & Goate, 2004). Sporadic AD, which may result from a variety of causal and contributing factors (genetic, environmental), afflicts 5–10% of individuals aged 65–74 years, 15–20% of those aged 75–84 years, and 40–50% of those aged 85 years and over; or a total of 4.5 million in the US today alone (Herbert *et al.*, 2003).

A common challenge for clinicians, primary care providers, and specialists alike, is recognizing the signs and symptoms of AD when a variety of other medical illnesses are present. In addition to increased risk for dementia, older adults are also at greater risk of a host of other health problems, including cardiovascular disease, hypertension, stroke, and so on, that are demanding of clinical attention. The typical 15-minute doctor–patient encounter may provide enough time for identifying and managing common physical health complaints, but not necessarily dementia. Persons with mild clinical AD often present as 'normal' in a brief encounter and are otherwise unlikely to acknowledge cognitive concerns. If the patient or family doesn't raise a concern about cognitive functional change and the clinician doesn't have the time or inclination to ask, care will remain focused primarily on physical health complaints. Under these conditions, dementia symptoms will eventually be recognized, but only later in the clinical progression when many more brain cells are likely to be dead or dying, thus complicating treatment.

The evaluative mindset

Clinicians with an *evaluative mindset* for AD demonstrate (1) awareness that older adults face a tangible and increasing risk for dementia with age; and (2) vigilance for cognitive functional changes atypical in the aging process alone, or in response to clinical depression. Whereas the average 65-year-old is relatively unlikely to have clinical AD or another form of dementing illness, the average 85-year-old, in contrast, faces a 1 in 2 chance. The clinician evaluating a patient in their eighties for the first time needs to consider the real possibility that AD (or another dementia) is present and investigate accordingly.

Part of this investigation is separating out what is normal for age and what is not. As shown in *Table 2.2*, how a patient reports a memory problem can provide clues (with other data) as to what may be going on[1]. Persons experiencing normal age-associated memory impairment may comment about not remembering as well as in the past but, for them, there is no functional loss. In normal aging, an item may be forgotten or unavailable for recall in an immediate sense, but the memory trace remains and is eventually recalled. For example, one may lose the car keys for a short period, but one eventually finds them. In contrast, in dementia, if a

Table 2.2 Memory complaints in normal aging, depression, and dementia

	Normal aging	*Depression*	*Clinical AD/dementia*
Complaint	May report a mild or subtle memory problem	More likely to complain about memory problems – 'I'm having terrible problems with my memory'	Expresses variable, nonspecific memory complaints – 'I forget sometimes' Or, may show little or no awareness of a memory problem –'I'm fine'
Functional interference	The problem does not interfere with daily functioning	Reported problems may interfere with daily functioning, but only minimally. Functional problems are more likely attributable to the mood disorder (lack of motivation, apathy, lethargy)	Clearly interferes with daily functioning (repeating the same questions or comments, missing appointments, forgetting to take medications on time, not paying bills appropriately or double paying them)
Cognitive status	Onset of the problem is unclear. Cognition normal on testing	Onset may be reported as sudden or abrupt. Subtle deficits may be apparent on testing, but these do not fit a typical dementia pattern	Gradual onset and progression. Cognition impaired on testing with gradual decline observed over time
Mood	Not associated with significant depressive or anxiety symptoms	Often associated with depressed or anxious mood	May be associated with fluctuating or blunted affect. Less likely to acknowledge overt depression, but a mood disorder may be present and contributing

(Adapted from Anstey & Low, 2004.)

[1] This paragraph simplifies the distinction between impairment stemming from normal aging, dementia, and depression. A whole book could be written about such distinctions. It is important for clinicians to consider these processes when evaluating a patient and make a best determination, based on available evidence, as to which may be involved. This determination may change over time as more evidence becomes available.

person loses the car keys, they do not recall where they are over time and it is just a chance occurrence if they find them. Persons with dementia typically do not complain of cognitive problems, others do. Family members notice functional changes and, as noted above, may raise the first red flag to the clinician or other health provider. Finally, persons with clinical depression may present as forgetful and even complain quite vehemently about memory loss, but their concerns are less likely to be corroborated by family reports and/or cognitive test results. It is important to note that these factors, aging, dementia, and depression can also co-exist and contribute together to observed impairment.

Change from baseline

When clinical AD is suspected, there are a number of ways to make a determination that impairment is truly present. A common strategy used in psychometric/cognitive testing is to compare an individual's observed performance with normative data from other like individuals (i.e. same gender, similar age, same level of education). Most tests of cognitive functioning, when administered to large samples of individuals, yield an inverted U or bell shaped curve (**2.1**). When plotted, many scores cluster around a mean or mid-point, with fewer scores at each end or 'tail' of the distribution. Scores at the high end, two standard deviations above the mean, may represent above average or superior performance, whereas those at the low end, two standard deviations below the mean, may be viewed as below average or indicative of significant impairment.

For the sake of discussion, let us assume that patient A, suspected of having dementia, scores in the below average range (one standard deviation below the mean) on a test for memory of a short story. From a psychometric standpoint, patient A would be viewed as having an objective deficit in memory only if A's score fell two standard deviations below what would be expected based on gender, age, and education norms. If A *should* have performed in the above average range because of high educational attainment (i.e. one standard deviation above the mean), but now scores in the below average range, this would be evidence consistent with a memory deficit and suggestive of a possible dementia process (assuming the support of other evaluative data).

An alternative to the psychometric approach is to characterize changes in cognitive functional status based on an *individual* determination. The early symptoms of clinical

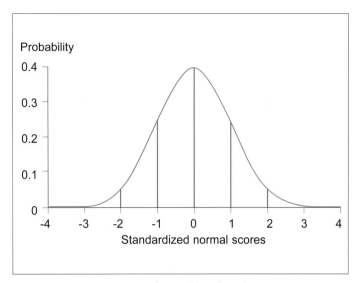

2.1 Normal distribution of cognitive function.

AD can be subtle and may not be evident in psychometric test performance. A person with high educational attainment, for example, can still score in the average range and yet also be starting to dement. A change-from-baseline approach allows the clinician to ask 'Is this individual functioning differently now from how he/she did 5–10 years ago?' and seek answers through history provided by patient and family. For example, let's say that patient B presents with a 1–2 year history of memory changes, but is still living independently and requires only minor assistance from family members to get by. B reports a problem, but denies that it is significant. His psychometric test scores are in the average, unimpaired range. His daughter, in contrast, reports a substantial change in functional status from just a few years ago 'He used to build intricate wooden models in the basement, but stopped because he can no longer remember well enough to execute the many steps involved. He can still do other simple things just fine, but not complex tasks like making models. This is a real change for him.' Such a report, in combination with other evidence, would be suggestive of a dementing process under a change-from-baseline approach. It is this approach, supplemented by psychometric/cognitive test scores when appropriate, that the authors advocate and will discuss for the remainder of this chapter.

In-office screening, interviewing, and staging

'The best diagnostic test is a careful history and physical and mental status examination by a physician with knowledge of and interest in dementia and the dementing diseases. Such an evaluation is time consuming, but nothing can replace it' (NIH Consensus Statement, 1987, p. 3413).

A simple flow chart for in-office assessment is shown in **2.2**. The first step is to determine a need for dementia-related evaluation. Is there evidence from patient or family report of a cognitive functional problem? If so, a focused interview with patient and a family informant would be warranted. What changes have been observed? In what areas of

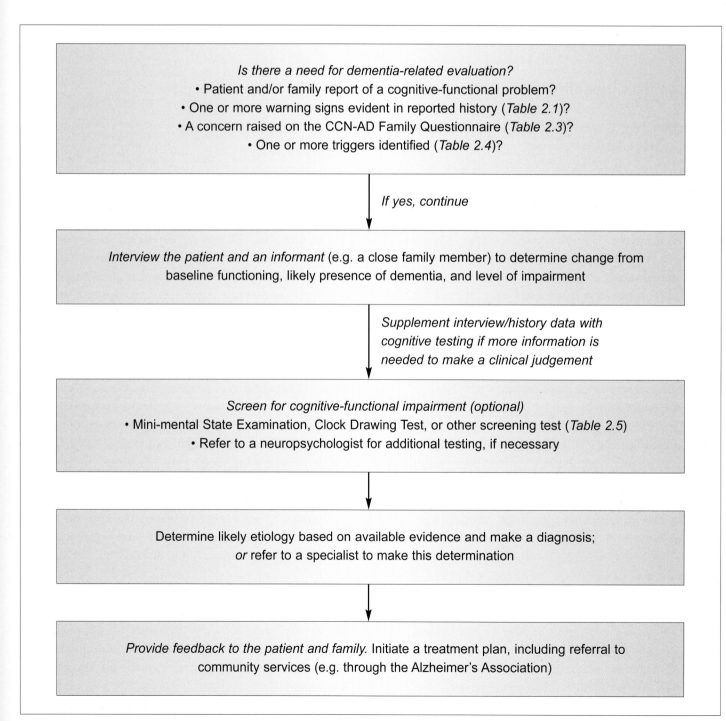

Is there a need for dementia-related evaluation?
• Patient and/or family report of a cognitive-functional problem?
• One or more warning signs evident in reported history (*Table 2.1*)?
• A concern raised on the CCN-AD Family Questionnaire (*Table 2.3*)?
• One or more triggers identified (*Table 2.4*)?

If yes, continue

Interview the patient and an informant (e.g. a close family member) to determine change from baseline functioning, likely presence of dementia, and level of impairment

Supplement interview/history data with cognitive testing if more information is needed to make a clinical judgement

Screen for cognitive-functional impairment (optional)
• Mini-mental State Examination, Clock Drawing Test, or other screening test (*Table 2.5*)
• Refer to a neuropsychologist for additional testing, if necessary

Determine likely etiology based on available evidence and make a diagnosis; *or* refer to a specialist to make this determination

Provide feedback to the patient and family. Initiate a treatment plan, including referral to community services (e.g. through the Alzheimer's Association)

2.2 Flow chart for in-office assessment for dementia.

cognition and/or function? For how long? Are there specific examples? Are the observed problems static or getting progressively worse? The Alzheimer's Association's 10 Warning Signs (*Table 2.1*), the Chronic Care Networks for Alzheimer's Disease (CCN-AD) Family Questionnaire (*Table 2.3*), and the Agency for Health Care Policy and Research's dementia evaluation 'triggers' (*Table 2.4*) can be helpful guides to the clinician in this interviewing process. Any of these tools could also be provided to a family informant as a waiting room questionnaire and then used as a point of reference during the interview process.

If, in the opinion of the clinician, there is reasonable evidence from this initial discussion that a dementing disorder is present, psychometric/cognitive testing may be pursued to gather more information (if necessary), or a more detailed evaluation may be initiated to obtain a diagnosis. *Table 2.5* lists a number of available cognitive screening measures for brief, in-office assessment. The Mini-mental State Examination (MMSE) is the most widely used

screening test. Others more specific to AD and other dementias include the Short Blessed Test (SBT) and General Practitioner Assessment of Cognition (GP-COG). Which screening measure a clinician chooses is often a matter of personal preference and experience. With all screening measures, however, it is important not to place too much confidence in a single score. False-positives and negatives are possible. The MMSE, for example, has a maximum score of 30 points, but the normal range can vary from the low 20s and up, depending on characteristics of the individual and testing situation. Low education and minority group membership are two factors that require attention in interpretation of lower scores. A score in the impaired range may not indicate true impairment for individuals from certain groups. Cognitive test scores, such as those derived from the MMSE, can inform and help verify a clinical impression based on interview and history data (i.e. using a change-from-baseline approach), but are never sufficient to determine dementia status alone.

Table 2.3 CCN-AD Family Questionnaire

In your opinion does _____ have problems with any of the following?

	Not at all	Sometimes	Frequently	Not applicable
1. Repeating or asking the same thing over and over?	0	1	2	
2. Remembering appointments, family occasions, holidays?	0	1	2	
3. Writing checks, paying bills, balancing the checkbook?	0	1	2	
4. Shopping independently (e.g. for clothing, groceries)?	0	1	2	
5. Taking medication according to instructions?	0	1	2	
6. Getting lost while walking or driving in familiar locations?	0	1	2	

Relationship to patient:

Total score:

According to CCN-AD guidelines, a total score of 3 or more should prompt the consideration of a more detailed evaluation. (Adapted from CCN-AD, 2003)

Table 2.4 Triggers for dementia evaluation

Does the person have increasing difficulty with any of the activities listed below?

Problem observed? Yes/No	Cognitive functional area
__Y __N	Learning and retaining new information: Is repetitive; has trouble remembering recent conversations, events, appointments; frequently misplaces objects
__Y __N	Handling complex tasks: Has trouble following a complex train of thought or performing tasks that require many steps such as balancing a checkbook or cooking a meal
__Y __N	Reasoning ability: Is unable to respond with a reasonable plan to problems at work or home, such as knowing what to do if the bathroom is flooded; shows uncharacteristic disregard for rules of social conduct
__Y __N	Spatial ability and orientation: Has trouble driving, organizing objects around the house, finding his or her way around familiar places
__Y __N	Language: Has increasing difficulty with finding the words to express what he or she wants to say and with following conversations
__Y __N	Behavior: Appears more passive and less responsive; is more irritable than usual; is more suspicious than usual; misinterprets visual or auditory stimuli

One or more positive (yes) responses would suggest a need for further evaluation to determine a possible cause or diagnosis.
(Adapted from Costa et al., 1996)

A detailed interview with the patient and a knowledgeable family member is the central process for dementia detection and diagnosis. A thorough medical history (including questions about cognitive functional status, past and present) coupled with an opportunity to corroborate information with an informant is typically required. This can be time consuming. The clinician must decide how much information is reasonable to obtain for a given patient and relative to other practice and reimbursement-related constraints.

At Washington University, the authors rely on the Clinical Dementia Rating (CDR) interview and scoring table to obtain and quantify information from the identified patient and a family informant (Hughes et al., 1982; Morris, 1993). The CDR is a 5-point scale used to characterize six domains of cognitive and functional performance applicable to Alzheimer's disease and related dementias: memory, orientation, judgment and problem solving, community affairs, home and hobbies, and personal care. The necessary information to make each rating is obtained through a semi-structured interview of the patient and a reliable informant.

The CDR table provides descriptive anchors that guide the clinician in making appropriate ratings based on available data and clinical judgment. In addition to ratings for each domain, an overall CDR score may be calculated through the use of an algorithm. This overall score is useful for characterizing and tracking a patient's level of impairment, and may be useful when giving diagnostic feedback to patient and family. CDR scores break down as follows:

0 = normal cognitive functioning (age-related changes only)
0.5 = very mild dementia
1 = mild dementia
2 = moderate dementia
3 = severe dementia

Table 2.5 Screening and staging measures

Measure	Notes
Brief screening tests	
Mini-mental State Examination (MMSE)	19 items measuring orientation, memory, concentration, language, and praxis; requires some test materials; ~10 minutes to administer; the most widely used screening test (Folstein *et al.*, 1975)
Short Blessed Test (SBT)	Six-item weighted version of the Information Memory Concentration Test (Blessed, *et al.*, 1968) ~5 minutes to administer; also correlated with Alzheimer's histopathology (Katzman *et al.*, 1983). A version developed through the Washington University Memory and Aging Project may be downloaded from http://alzheimer.wustl.edu.
General Practitioner Assessment of Cognition (GP-COG)	Includes a six-item screening test similar to the SBT, a clock drawing task, and a five-item informant questionnaire; ~10 minutes to administer (Brodaty *et al.*, 2002)
7 Minute Screen	Four tests (orientation, memory, clock drawing, and verbal fluency); ~7–10 minutes to administer (Solomon & Pendlebury, 1998)
Clinical Staging Instruments (global measures of dementia severity)	
Clinical Dementia Rating (CDR)	Five-point ordinal scale; assesses cognitive and functional abilities by a structured informant interview and patient testing in 6 domains with descriptors for each level of severity (Hughes *et al.*, 1982; Morris, 1993)
Global Deterioration Scale (GDS)	Seven-point ordinal scale; has global descriptors for each severity level; a 35-item Brief Cognitive Rating Scale (BCRS) assists in assignment of the global rating (Reisberg *et al.*, 1982)

(Adapted from Buckles *et al.*, 2000)

Information about the CDR and training options for its use may be accessed on-line at http://alzheimer.wustl.edu/cdr. A number of other diagnostic and staging guides for AD are available through journal articles and on-line. Here is a partial list:

American Academy of Neurology – Practice Parameters – *Diagnosis of Dementia* (Knopman *et al.*, 2001); *Early Detection of Dementia: Mild Cognitve Impairment* (Petersen *et al.*, 2001). Available on-line at http://www.aan.com/publications/practice/ index.cfm

Chronic Care Networks for Alzheimer's Disease – *Tools for Early Identification, Assessment, and Treatment* (http://www.nccconline.org/about/alzheimers.htm)

Alzheimer's Association – On-line Catalog of Assessment Tools and Resources (http://www.alz.org/Resources/TopicIndex/Diagnosis.asp #assessment)

Differential diagnosis

Once it is determined that a dementing disorder is present and at what stage (very mild, mild, and so on), it is important for treatment to identify a likely cause. Clinical AD is the most common dementing illness in older age (i.e. after age 65 years) and should be considered first. In its early stages, clinical AD is primarily a disorder of memory. Long-standing, remote memories remain intact, while recent memory is failing. Persons with early clinical AD forget appointments, misplace items, repeat questions or comments in conversation, and have difficulty managing finances and other complex tasks with high memory demands. As time goes on, problems handling multi-part tasks become apparent, language deficits (both receptive and/or expressive) appear, and disorientation occurs. In time, recent memory failure gives way to more pervasive problems in recall. Even long-standing memories from decades ago become patchy and eventually fade altogether as the disease moves from moderate to severe levels. Personality change (notably withdrawal) and depressed mood can also occur during progression.

Although some dementia cases will present in this 'classic' pattern, many will not. Another less common neurodegenerative disease may be the cause of observed symptoms. AD neuropathology may also co-exist with one or more other dementing pathologies, each contributing to the clinical picture. Some primary care clinicians may choose to refer to a specialist (i.e. neurologist, psychiatrist, geriatrician) when faced with a complex case. Alternatively, some may choose to make a provisional diagnosis based on available information and seek to confirm this over time. *Table 2.6* presents a simplified listing of symptoms atypical for AD and other diseases to consider in differential diagnosis. For example, AD patients rarely experience vivid visual hallucinations, yet this symptom is quite common in dementia with Lewy bodies. The disease-specific chapters in this book provide detailed information on presenting symptoms and differential diagnosis from AD.

Table 2.6 Differential diagnosis considerations for unusual features

Symptom/feature	Consideration for differential diagnosis
Abrupt onset	Vascular dementia
Stepwise deterioration	Vascular dementia
Prominent behavioral changes	Frontotemporal dementia
Profound apathy	Frontotemporal dementia
Prominent aphasia	Frontotemporal dementia; vascular dementia
Progressive gait disorder	Vascular dementia; hydrocephalus
Prominent fluctuations in level of consciousness or cognitive abilities	Delirium due to infection, medications, or other causes; dementia with Lewy bodies; seizures
Hallucinations or delusions	Delirium due to infection, medications, or other causes; dementia with Lewy bodies
Extrapyramidal signs or gait disturbance	Parkinsonian syndromes; vascular dementia
Eye-movement abnormalities	Progressive supranuclear palsy; Wernicke's encephalopathy

(Adapted from Kawas, 2003)

Engaging the family and community referral sources

A common 'mistake' in clinical dementia care is choosing not to engage family members in the diagnosis and management process. This may occur in response to a specific patient request ('I don't want my family to know that I have a memory problem'), a concern about breaking confidentiality (e.g. relative to the Health Insurance Portability and Accountability Act [HIPAA] confidentiality law in the US), a reluctance to complicate the care situation by involving other parties, or another legitimate concern. Whatever the reason, once diagnosed with a dementing disorder, a patient is at increasing risk of negative outcomes over time. The patient may forget to take medications on time or at all; the patient may forget that driving privileges were suspended and continue to drive; the patient may fall victim to telemarketers or mail order scams and forfeit needed resources, and so on. Family members are typically (though not always) in the best position to monitor, guide, and protect persons with AD over time. It is usually best to find a way to communicate with and involve family in the care process whenever possible.

Referral to community services and resources can also be extremely helpful to families. In the US, the Alzheimer's Association provides informational support, respite care, and case management services, 24-hour helpline assistance, and support groups for the benefit of persons with dementia and family members alike. Area Agencies on Aging are another source of information and supportive services in many US cities. Similar organizations exist in other countries. The more resources and services a family can muster, the better their chances to cope effectively in the provision of dementia care over time.

Case example

John Doe is a 78-year-old, retired postal worker, with 12 years of education. He lives with his wife of 47 years, Doris, in a 2-bedroom home in small city in central US. Mr Doe and his wife have one child, a son, Paul, who lives 300 miles away. Paul is married with three children and manages a construction business. He is close to his parents emotionally, but rarely has time to visit or otherwise assist them. Mr Doe, a Korean War veteran, retired at age 65 years and spends a few days per week volunteering at the local Veterans of Foreign Wars (VFW) Hall. He is active at church and enjoys playing golf 2–3 times per week.

Over the past 18 months, Mrs Doe has become increasingly concerned about her husband's memory for recent events and information. He repeats himself regularly and has forgotten to follow through on commitments, only to deny later that he ever knew about them. At first, she attributed some of this behavior to his cantankerous personality – he just doesn't care about things as he used to – but her level of concern increased when he forgot his way home from the VFW Hall and drove for an hour before becoming oriented again. She convinced him to see his doctor following this incident on a pretense (a shoulder injury sustained while mowing the lawn needed attention), but with the intention of asking about his memory loss at the same time.

During the appointment with his primary care physician, Mr Doe acknowledged having some 'slight forgetfulness' but downplayed its significance. 'I'm getting older and I don't need to keep track of things as in the past. I'm doing just fine.' His physician, Dr Roberts, asked about depression or other stresses in his life. 'I have no such problems' was the reply. This was later confirmed by his wife. He also asked about history of memory loss in Mr Doe's family (his mother showed signs of dementia in her late 70s but was never diagnosed) and then decided to administer the MMSE. Mr Doe scored 23 of 30 points, missing items in orientation (incorrect month, date, and floor of the building), mental control (two errors in counting backwards by 7), and memory (only recalled 1 of 3 words after a brief delay).

Mr Doe was clearly surprised by his performance, but also somewhat incredulous: 'I'm sure I'll do better on that next time.'

Dr Roberts asked to speak with Mrs Doe separately and Mr Doe agreed. During this 5-minute interview, Mrs Doe told of her husband getting lost and an important commitment at the VFW Hall that he completely forgot. 'I've never known him to get lost or forget something like this. I'm really worried for him. I recall his mother having similar problems, but only now am I connecting things.' She reported that his memory was getting gradually worse over time. This information convinced Dr Roberts to order an MRI brain scan and laboratory tests to rule out an acute or reversible cause for his apparent cognitive dysfunction.

All medical tests and scans came back normal. Based on Mrs Doe's convincing report of gradual decline, and Mr Doe's errors on the MMSE, particularly in memory and orientation (two areas affected early in the course of clinical AD), Dr Roberts chose to make a diagnosis of probable mild AD and initiated drug therapy. He planned to follow Mr Doe closely and confirm this diagnostic impression over time.

Neither of the Does seemed surprised by the diagnosis, although Mr Doe didn't seem particularly concerned either. Mrs Doe expressed relief to 'finally know' why her husband was having problems. Dr Roberts referred them both to the Alzheimer's Association for education and support group assistance. He encouraged Mr Doe to continue in as many volunteer and other activities as he felt comfortable, but also asked Mrs Doe to monitor her husband's activities more closely. As a precaution, given that Mr Doe had become lost while driving, Dr Roberts also asked him to restrict his driving to daylight hours and familiar areas for now (thinking that a driving evaluation for safety reasons may be required sometime over the next year). A follow-up appointment was set up for 6 months hence.

Comment

The case of Mr Doe represents a fairly typical presentation of mild clinical AD: (1) memory loss and disorientation were gradually becoming a problem; (2) depression or unusual symptoms were not evident; (3) his wife reported clear examples of uncharacteristic failings; (4) there was a family history of dementia in his mother; and (5) he scored in the impaired range on a widely used screening test with errors consistent with historic report. This information was enough for Dr Roberts to make a diagnosis of probable mild AD and initiate drug therapy. His recommendations to stay active, monitor more closely, get involved with the Alzheimer's Association, begin restricting driving were consistent with Mr Doe's history and provided a structure for management in the future. Follow-up in 6 months would give Dr Roberts an opportunity to re-administer the MMSE, check on Mr Doe's response to medication, and lay the groundwork for future care.

With regards to driving and dementia, the American Academy of Neurology recommends that persons with mild dementia (CDR 1 level) stop driving for safety reasons (Dubinsky *et al.*, 2000). Dr Roberts is clearly aware of this recommendation, but chooses not to 'hit' the Does with it right away. Rather, he suggests a prudent restriction in driving exposure and lays the groundwork to revisit this issue in the coming months.

References

Alzheimer's Association (2004). 10 Warning Signs of Alzheimer's Disease. An on-line publication of the Alzheimer's Association: (http://www.alz.org/AboutAD/Warning.asp).

American Psychiatric Association (1994). *Diagnostic and Statistical Manual of Mental Disorders* (4th edn.). American Psychiatric Association, Washington.

Anstey KJ, Low LF (2004). Normal cognitive changes in aging. *Aus. Family Phys.* **33**:783–787.

Blessed G, Tomlinson BE, Roth M (1968). The association between quantitative measures of dementia and of senile change in the cerebral grey matter of elderly subjects. *Br. J. Psych.* **114**:797–811.

Brodaty H, Pond D, Kemp NM, *et al.* (2002). The GPCOG: a new screening test for dementia designed for general practice. *J. Am. Geriatric Soc.* **50**:530–534.

Buckles VD, Coats M, Morris JC (2000). *Best Practice of Medicine: Dementia.* Merck Medicus (http://merck.micromedex.com)

Chronic Care Networks for Alzheimer's Disease (2003). *Tools for early identification, assessment and treatment for people with Alzheimer's disease and dementia.* A publication of the Alzheimer's Association and National Chronic Care Consortium (http://www.alz.org/Resources/FactSheets/CCN-AD03.pdf; page 9).

Connell CM, Janevic MR, Gallant MP (2001). The costs of caring: impact of dementia on family caregivers. *J. Geriatric Psych. Neurol.* **14**(4):179–187.

Costa PT, *et al.* (1996). *Clinical Practice Guideline, Quick Reference Guide for Clinicians* (No. 19), US Department of Health and Human Services, Rockville.

Davis P (2004). *The Long Goodbye: Memories of My Father.* Alfred A Knopf Publishing, New York.

DeBaggio T (2002). *Losing My Mind: An Intimate Look at Life with Alzheimer's,* The Free Press/Simon & Schuster, New York.

Dubinsky RM, Stein AC, Lyons K (2000). Practice parameter: risk of driving and Alzheimer's disease (an evidence-based review): Report of the Quality Standards Subcommittee of the American Academy of Neurology. *Neurology* **54**:2205–2211.

Folstein MF, *et al.* (1975). *J. Psych. Res.* **12**:189–198.

Hebert LE, Scherr PA, Bienias JL, *et al.* (2003). Alzheimer's disease in the US population: prevalence estimates using the 2000 census. *Arch. Neurol.* **60**:1119–1122.

Hughes CP, Berg L, Danziger WL, *et al.* (1982). A new clinical scale for the staging of dementia. *Br. J. Psych.* **140**:566–572.

Katzman R, Brown T, Fuld P, Peck A, Schechter R, Schimmel H (1983). Validation of a short Orientation-Memory-Concentration test of cognitive impairment. *Am. J. Psych.* **140**:734–739.

Kawas CH (2003). Early Alzheimer's disease. *N. Engl. J. Med.* **349**:1056–1063.

Keefover RW (1990). Alzheimer's disease as a diagnosis of exclusion. *W. Virginia Med. J.* **86**(2):51–55.

Knopman DS, DeKosky ST, Cummings JL, *et al.* (2001). Practice parameter: diagnosis of dementia (an evidence-based review). Report of the Quality Standards Subcommittee of the American Academy of Neurology. *Neurology* **56**(9):1143–1153.

Meuser TM, Boise L, Morris JC (2004). Clinician beliefs and practice in dementia care: implications for health educators. *Ed. Geront.* **30**:491–516.

Marwit SJ, Meuser TM (2002). Development and initial validation of an inventory to assess grief in caregivers of persons with Alzheimer's disease. *Gerontologist* **42**(6):751–765.

Meuser TM, Marwit SJ (2001). A comprehensive, stage-sensitive model of grief in dementia caregiving. *Gerontologist* **41**(5):658–700.

Morris JC (1993). The Clinical Dementia Rating (CDR): current version and scoring rules. *Neurology* **43**:2412–2414.

Murphy DD, Ravina B (2003). Brain banking for neurodegenerative diseases. *Curr. Opin. Neurol.* **16**(4):459–463.

National Institutes of Health (1987). Differential diagnosis of dementing diseases: NIH Consensus Statement. *JAMA* **258**(23):3411–3416.

Pastor P, Goate AM (2004). Molecular genetics of Alzheimer's disease. *Curr. Psych. Reports* **6**(2):125–133.

Petersen RC, Stevens JC, Ganguli M, *et al.* (2001). Practice parameter: early detection of dementia: mild cognitive impairment (an evidence-based review). Report of the Quality Standards Subcommittee of the American Academy of Neurology. *Neurology* **56**(9):1133–1142.

Reisberg B, Ferris SH, de Leon MJ, *et al.* (1982). Global Deterioration Scale. *Am. J. Psych.* **139**:1136–1139.

Small GW, Rabins PV, Barry PP, *et al.* (1997). Diagnosis and treatment of Alzheimer disease and related disorders. Consensus statement of the American Association for Geriatric Psychiatry, the Alzheimer's Association, and the American Geriatrics Society. *JAMA* **278**:1363–1371.

Solomon PR, Pendlebury WW (1998). Recognition of Alzheimer's disease: the 7 Minute Screen. *Family Med.* **30**:265–271.

Diagnosis of Alzheimer's disease: neuropathologic investigation methods

Introduction

This chapter describes protocols used to establish definitive pathological diagnoses using autopsy central nervous system (CNS) material from demented subjects. The presentation is divided into four parts: (1) the autopsy procedures for obtaining brain, spinal cord, cerebrospinal fluid (CSF), and pituitary gland specimens; (2) the diagnostic algorithm used to distinguish brains with healthy aging changes from those with pure or mixed dementing disorders; and (3) the histologic and immunohistochemical (IHC) methods that were used in Washington University's Alzheimer's Disease Research Center (ADRC) from 1986 to 2004 in order to assign final neuropathologic diagnoses on primary and secondary causes of dementia. Part 4 describes emerging diagnostic methods that materially add to knowledge of pathogenic mechanisms of dementing disorders.

Establishing a histopathologic baseline for normality is a necessary task in order to assess the presence or absence of the burgeoning multiplicity of dementing diseases, which is the main focus of Part 2. In the case of nondemented controls, the primary goals of postmortem brain examination are to study: (1) any incidental pathologic changes; (2) brain lesions due to aging *per se*, and (3) to assess the possible presence of preclinical pathologic aging-related Alzheimer's disease (AD). The specific neuropathologic findings associated with these three categories of changes in cognitively intact control brains are more fully described in Chapters 4 and 5.

Part 3 provides a practical rationale the ADRC uses for specific dye and immunohistochemical techniques used to study the healthy aging brain and to diagnose AD and the non-AD dementing disorders and their preclinical forms.

Removing and processing the brain, spinal cord, pituitary gland, and cerebrospinal fluid at autopsy

Autopsy protocol

The following protocols are those required by the state of Missouri, US. Since 1999, mentally competent persons have been able to sign their own autopsy permits. Separate autopsy permission from family members after death is not necessary. Other persons must have an autopsy permit signed after death by the legal next-of-kin according to a hierarchy of relationships (e.g. from the Missouri autopsy statutes, website URL: http://www.moga.state.mo.us/statutes/C100-199/1940000115.htm). Research subjects whose brain or other postmortem tissues or bodily fluids will be used for genetic analyses must also agree to and sign a Genetics Consent document that is approved by the Institutional Review Board (IRB). Genetic analyses related to dementing disorders might include apolipoprotein E (apoE) allele genotyping of DNA, or DNA sequencing to define etiologic mutations for AD (Bertram & Tanzi, 2004), Parkinson's disease (PD) (Forman *et al.*, 2005a), or various tauopathies (Rademakers *et al.*, 2004).

Reviewing clinical data

The clinical history available to the neuropathologist at the time of death includes the following: (1) current and past hospital medical charts; (2) information on the 'Clinical Abstract' portion of the autopsy permission form that includes the suspected clinical cause/s of death and any special features that need to be investigated; (3) information from the postmortem dementia assessment conducted by ADRC nurse coordinators; and (4) research information contained in an on-line 'Autopsy Database'. The latter ADRC-wide resource, a subset of information in the main SAS Institute, Cary, NC database, is accessed over secure virtual private network connections that utilize a user identity, password, and data encryption to comply with Health Insurance Portability and Accountability Act regulations. The Autopsy Database information includes: the Clinical Dementia Rating (CDR) (Hughes *et al.*, 1982; Morris, 1993) or CDR at the last clinical assessment; the year of dementia onset (from which the total duration of dementia can be readily calculated); the final clinical diagnoses of the underlying cause/s of dementia; the date, place and time of death; and known current medications. The postmortem interval (PMI) can then be calculated as the time interval in fractional hours (e.g. 9.2) that elapsed between pronouncement of death and CSF or brain tissue collection and storage at -80°C or fixation in 10% (commercial) neutral buffered formalin (10% NBF). Criteria are currently being finalized by several national committees to define a standard set of agonal factors to be recorded by all ADRCs at the time of death (see Appendix for details of the National Alzheimer's Coordinating Center [NACC]). The ADRC Neuropathology Core Leaders and their Quality Assurance and Standards subcommittee are considering standard methods to assess brain tissue integrity at the time of death. Such measures might include assessment of brain pH and Western blot analysis to assess messenger ribonucleic acid (mRNA) yield and quality (Kingsbury *et al.*, 1995).

Postmortem CSF, brain and pituitary removal and processing

At the time of autopsy a scalpel is used to incise the scalp, being careful to reflect the skull and not cut the hair. A reciprocating saw is used to detach the dome of the skull and a triangular notch is cut in the frontal bone to stabilize the position of the 'skull cap' once it is replaced. Both outer and inner surfaces of the dura are inspected after being 'stripped' by the autopsy assistants. Any sites of bleeding, trauma to the scalp and soft tissues, or skull fractures are recorded on autopsy forms. This part of the brain examination is important, particularly in elderly persons who are either at risk for falling or have fallen (often many times). Falls are common in AD and dementia with Lewy body (DLB) patients in particular. The brain is then accessible for CSF collection, brain and pituitary removal, frozen tissue collection, and chemical fixation.

Postmortem CSF collection

The falx cerebri is removed with scissors and forceps and the the two medial surfaces of the cerebral hemispheres are gently separated to expose the junction of the anterior and middle thirds of the corpus callosum (CC), the target site for withdrawing CSF (**3.1**). One hand is stabilized by resting firmly on the frontal bone and the beveled needle tip of a sterile, disposable long spinal tap needle is inserted just

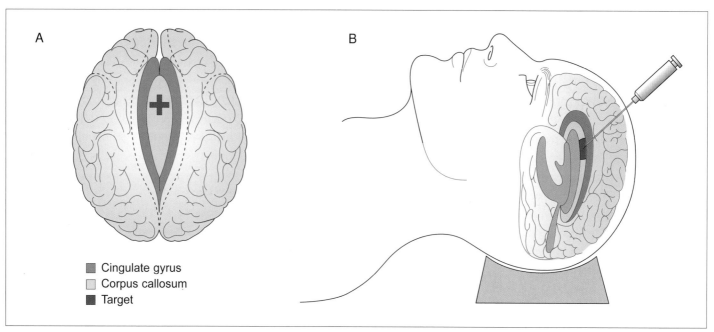

3.1 A Location for withdrawing cerebrospinal fluid at autopsy from the exposed cerebrum after removing the skull cap. The needle, positioned as shown in (**B**), is inserted at the junction of the exposed anterior 1/3 and posterior 2/3rds of the corpus callosum at a 45° angle. The bevel of the needle is just below the inferior border of the corpus callosum.

beneath the CC. The goal is to withdraw 30 ml of CSF. Obtaining this amount of fluid is often possible in moderately and severely demented persons with advanced cerebral atrophy and dilated cerebral ventricles. However, experience with over 300 nondemented and demented autopsy cases indicates that the amount of CSF obtained with the initial attempt is usually all that is possible. Further attempts at collecting additional CSF volume often lead to outright failure, or obtaining CSF contaminated with blood or brain tissue fragments. Failures on 'second attempt' CSF collection from cadavers is due either to the cerebral ventricles not being enlarged or to collapse of the ventricles during CSF removal. Collected postmortem CSF (pmCSF) is first placed in a 100 ml sterile plastic urine cup on ice. Aliquots (2 ml) are then placed into 15 prelabeled, screw-capped, low temperature cryotubes and frozen at -80°C without further treatment. The volume and clarity of the collected pmCSF is recorded on a standard data form.

As far as use of pmCSF for clinicopathologic research, initial experiments have shown that postmortem proteolysis causes severe artifactual elevations in phosphorylated tau in pmCSF, with four separate antibodies, that invalidates this measurement (Morihara *et al.*, 1998; DW McKeel, Jr & P Davies, unpublished data). On the other hand, measurement of pmCSF beta-amyloid levels may be possible as this protein appears to be more stable after death (Strozyk *et al.*, 2003).

Brain removal and initial processing for histologic examination, diagnostic and research IHC and biochemical analysis

Once pmCSF has been collected and placed on ice, the dural attachments along the lateral surfaces of the cerebral hemispheres and the tentorium cerebelli are detached using a number 11 (sharp pointed) scalpel blade, being careful to avoid incising the brain. Next the olfactory bulbs and tracts are dislodged gently from the cribriform plate and are reflected backwards for subsequent harvesting. The surgical scalpel and number 11 blade are used to cut both optic nerves at the optic foramina and to sever the internal carotid arteries (ICAs) as they exit the cavernous sinus on either side of the sella turcica containing the pituitary gland. Scissors occasionally may be required to cut through heavily calcified ICAs. Each cranial nerve is then cut as close to the skull base as possible. Once the tentorium has been incised and the brain stem exposed, the vertebral arteries can be identified and cut using a long-handled #3 scalpel handle with a number 11 blade. For 'brain only' limited brain autopsy cases especially, it is important to sever the spinal cord as far down in the foramen magnum as possible using the same instrument.

Examination of the spinal cord is frequently neglected in neurodegenerative disorders despite growing evidence in the literature that this structure is involved in several dementing disorders (Kato *et al.*, 1992; Holton *et al.*, 2001).

Removal of the entire spinal cord at autopsy

Using a standard anterior approach after the organ block has been removed, the anterior vertebral bodies are removed *en bloc* with a reciprocating saw. The cord and dura with attached dorsal and ventral nerve roots and dorsal root ganglia should be removed as a whole. The spinal dura should be opened along its entire length to allow removal of segments to be snap frozen and to allow uniform exposure of the cord to 10% NBF for optimal histopathologic examination.

Removal and fixation of the pituitary at autopsy

Once the brain has been removed, the dural diaphragma sellae is circumferentially incised with a number 11 scalpel blade on a #3 long handle to expose the hypophysis (pituitary gland). Smooth tipped forceps are used to grasp a dural edge and the gland is removed using gentle traction and sharp dissection. The gland is then bivalved in the mid-horizontal plane using a Pathco™ double edged surgical knife and blade after it is weighed to the tenth of a gram (**3.2**, overleaf). Normal mean pituitary weight obtained in this manner for adults is about 0.6–0.7 g with a range of 0.3–0.7 g being normal for elderly adults who die after 70 years of age. The gland halves are placed in a regular tissue cassette and fixed for 2 days in 10% NBF. Paraffin sections (5 μm) are examined with hematoxylin eosin (H&E) to visualize cytologic features of the stalk, neurohypophysis, 'invading adrenocorticotropic hormone (ACTH) basophils' of the posterior lobe, the glandular pars tuberalis surrounding the pituitary stalk, the pars intermedia residual Rathke pouch follicular glands, and the adenohypophyseal red eosinophil classic growth hormone-secreting acidophils, the classic ACTH-secreting basophils (high granular affinity for hematoxylin with a large vacuole), and secretory cells with poorly granulated, faintly staining cytoplasm, the classic anterior pituitary chromophobes (Fowler & McKeel, 1979a, b).

3.2 One-half of the pituitary gland sectioned in the mid-horizontal plane parallel to the skull base shows a central, gelatinous appearing adenoma. The surrounding adenohypophysis (AP) is a variegated orange color. The neurohypophysis (NP) is the elliptical white structure at the top center of the hypophysis. One large pars intermedia follicle is visible as a dark area between the center of the AP and the NP.

The rationale for examining the pituitary gland in dementia cases rests on the following data: (1) screening for hypothyroidism is frequently done to rule out this treatable and hence reversible cause of dementia. The anterior pituitary gland shows thyroid stimulating hormone (TSH) (thyrotrope) hypertrophy, hyperplasia, and adenoma formation in cases of untreated hypothyoidsim (Horvath *et al.*, 1999); (2) dopaminergic deficits (e.g. as occur in PD) may be reflected by release of tonic dopaminergic inhibition of anterior pituitary prolactin cells leading to prolactin cell hyperplasia and hyperprolactinemia (Bellomo *et al.*, 1991); and (3) systemic disorders that produce cardiovascular signs and symptoms all cause ischemic lesions in the pituitary gland. Some examples of these disorders include diabetes mellitus (Watson & Craft, 2003), myocardial infarction, bilateral carotid strokes, and head trauma.

Most endocrine system disorders are reflected in pituitary gland cytomorphology. This type of information may be a useful adjunct in assessing the degree of involvement of the endocrine hypothalamus when a dementing disorder affects this crucial brain region (e.g. AD where plaques and tangles are common). Corroboration of diabetes mellitus may be obtained by observing lymphocytes in the pars intermedia, ACTH hyperplasia, and scattered stellate ischemic scars

(healed microinfarcts) in the adenohypophysis. Such lesions are common in pituitary glands from insulin-requiring diabetics (see Appendix for details of National Diabetes Research Interchange [NDRI]) (Flynn *et al.*, 1988).

Examination of peripheral nerve and muscle tissue in dementia cases

The importance of examining clinically affected skeletal muscle and peripheral nerve in non-AD dementias cannot be overemphasized. The need to do so in classical lower motor neuron diseases (MND) with advanced muscle atrophy such as amyotrophic lateral sclerosis (ALS) is obvious. However, clinical signs of MND in frontotemporal dementia (FTD) disorders may be very subtle, initially consisting of muscle fasciculations detectable only by electromyographic methods and mild deficits in nerve conduction velocities (de Carvalho, 2001).

Morphologic data on spinal cord, peripheral nerves and skeletal muscle are sorely lacking in the FTD-MND disorders. Examination of skeletal muscle may be especially rewarding as some 'muscle diseases' show accumulation of the same two proteins, beta amyloid and hyperphosphory-lated tau, that characterize AD senile plaques and neurofibrillary tangles (Vattemi *et al.*, 2003). Muscle and nerve changes may be part of hereditary dementing disorders as well (fragile-X carriers) (Forman *et al.*, 2005b).

Autopsy techniques for examining skeletal muscle and peripheral nerve
Techniques for examining human sural nerve and skeletal muscle biopsies (Kanda *et al.*, 1996) may be applied to human postmortem specimens.

Examining peripheral nerve samples
Portions of the sural nerve should be frozen, placed in neutral buffered glutaraldehyde electron microscopy (EM) fixative, and a third segment fixed in 10% NBF for routine diagnostic evaluation. Nerve fiber 'tease' preparations are valuable for assessing segmental demyelinating processes and axonal loss, for example as occurs in diabetic neuropathy. Luxol fast blue-periodic acid-Schiff (PAS, the Klüver–Barrera stain; Klüver & Barrera, 1953; Luna, 1968) and impregnation with osmium tetroxide ('osmic acid') are useful for studying such preparations. Nerve specimens embedded in EM plastics, cut at 0.5–1.0 µm, and stained

with toluidine blue are highly informative for assessing both myelinated and unmyelinated nerve fibers at high resolution, fiber density, and size distribution at the light microscopic level. Schwann cells, fibroblasts, and inflammatory cells can be easily identified with greater diagnostic certainty than is the case for thicker paraffin sections.

Examining skeletal muscle samples

Skeletal muscle samples should include appropriate clinically-affected muscles. Autopsy muscle samples can be fixed in a muscle surgical biopsy clamp; however, good morphologic preservation still can be obtained if one is not available. Muscle samples, similar to peripheral nerve, should be fixed in 10% NBF for histopathologic examination. An additional muscle sample also should be snap frozen in liquid nitrogen to facilitate muscle immunohistochemistry and biochemistry. Both cross sections and longitudinal sections of skeletal muscle should be examined. This is required to detect subtle early changes. Plastic-embedded skeletal muscle specimens (1 μm) are useful for studying muscle fiber size and shape, fiber inclusions, and the nature of infiltrating cells. For example, subtle morphologic changes such as fiber angulation, a prelude to group fiber atrophy, help to diagnose early ALS–MND (Troost et al., 1992).

Washington University ADRC algorithm for diagnosing AD and non-AD dementias as distinct from healthy brain aging

Neuropathologists face several distinct challenges in assessing postmortem brains for a histopathologic diagnosis of AD. These hurdles include: (1) a lack of standardized criteria for diagnosing preclinical pathologic AD; (2) confusion in the literature between mild cognitive impairment (MCI) (Petersen, 2004) and very mild AD as defined by the CDR (McKeel et al., 1993; Kirshner, 2005); and (3) lack of comprehensive information about cognitive status near the time of death. Another difficulty is interpreting co-occurring dementing disorders such as small vascular infarcts with respect to their contribution to the overall degree of cognitive impairment.

This chapter will first consider each of these challenges and will emphasize diagnostically useful neuropathologic methods. It will then suggest an algorithmic approach to AD

diagnosis, developed to classify AD and co-occurring neurodegenerative disorders efficiently.

The algorithm currently used evolved from a diagnostic protocol for various dementing disorders that was proposed by Lowe (1998). Several reviews and monographs that cover the full spectrum of neurodegenerative disorders include those by Markesbery (1998), Esiri and colleagues (1997; 2004), and an International Society of Neuropathology monograph edited by Dickson (2003).

Figure **3.3** (overleaf) includes the diagnostic algorithm currently in use at the author's medical center and ADRC for classifying AD and non-AD dementing disorders. This scheme has evolved during the accession of more than 1,020 brains that were collected between 1981 and mid-2004. A number of studies have now been published (Crystal et al., 1988; Katzman et al., 1988; Morris et al., 1996) showing that a significant minority of clinically assessed nondemented persons have AD pathology on brain autopsy, now defined as 'preclinical pathologic AD'. There is some confusion about the use of the term 'preclinical' at both the clinical and pathologic levels. Some investigators apply preclinical only to persons whose cognition is completely intact (i.e. CDR 0), assessed by the most stringent methods including the use of a close collateral source. Other investigators use the term to refer to persons who do not meet formal Alzheimer's Disease and Related Disorders Association (ADRDA) (Blackwell et al., 2004) or DSM-III or -IV criteria for dementia, even though there are subtle cognitive impairments.

None of the existing standardized diagnostic methods based on histopathology are entirely adequate for diagnosing preclinical or very mild (CDR 0.5) pathologic AD. Cognitive profiles of a CDR 0.5 group of patients studied by the author overlap with individuals described in the literature as having MCI (Grundman et al., 2004; Desai & Grossberg, 2005). Indeed, 70% of CDR 0.5/MCI overlap patients progress to overt CDR 1 AD within 2 years (Goldman et al., 2001). Some key features that differentiate the three main diagnostic schemes for AD are presented in Table 3.1 (overleaf). For convenience in the following paragraphs the author will refer to total (diffuse and neuritic) senile plaques (TSP), diffuse senile plaques (DSP) and neuritic senile plaques (NSP).

3.3 Flow diagram to show the diagnostic schema followed at the author's center to make a pathologic diagnosis of specific dementing disorders. Alzheimer's disease is first ruled in or out, then Lewy diseases, then tauopathies, frontotemporal dementias and miscellaneous disorders, such as prion-related diseases.

Table 3.1 Neuropathologic diagnosis of Alzheimer's disease: 3 leading sets of criteria

Criteria	Age-adjusted	Main features	Citation
NIA-Khachaturian	Yes	Neocortex total plaques (diffuse and neuritic)	Khachaturian (1985)
CERAD	Yes	Cortex neuritic plaques only	Mirra *et al.* (1991)
NIA–Reagan Institute	No	Neuritic plaques only; Braak NFP staging	NIA–Reagan (1997); Braak and Braak (1991)

CERAD: Consortium to Establish a Registry for Alzheimer's Disease; NFP: neurofibrillary pathology (tangles, neuropil threads, senile plaque neurites)

The National Institute on Aging (NIA) (Khachaturian, 1985) criteria

The National Institute on Aging (NIA) (Khachaturian, 1985) criteria are based on the age-adjusted density (number per mm^2) of diffuse and neuritic senile plaques (TSP) in any area of the prefrontal, temporal, parietal, or medial occipital neocortex. These criteria are the only ones that are quantitative. The higher the age at death, the higher the threshold for plaque density (*Table 3.2*). The presence of some neocortical tangles is required up to age 75 years but not thereafter. A built-in feature (often overlooked) is thus recognition of the fact that overall plaque and tangle burden may be less in the very elderly, a point that has been established by independent studies (Giannakopoulos et al., 1996; Berg et al., 1998).

Currently, the original Khachaturian 1985 NIA consensus criteria have been supplanted by the newer NIA-Reagan Institute criteria (1997). The primary reasons for this included a feeling among some investigators that plaque quantification was too difficult reliably across CERAD diagnostic centers (Mirra et al., 1994). Also, the 1997 NIA-Reagan Working Group believed that the addition of tangle-based scoring using the Braak and Braak (1991a) system would add to the usefulness of the criteria. A recent study, building on previous Washington University ADRC data (McKeel et al., 1993), showed that modified Khachaturian diagnostic criteria provide the highest available sensitivity and specificity for distinguishing between pure (i.e. no co-morbid dementing disorders) nondemented cognitively normal CDR 0 controls and pure clinical AD (McKeel et al., 2004).

The Consortium to Establish a Registry for Diagnosing AD (CERAD) criteria

This North American consortium of 28 participating Alzheimer centers developed a new set of pathologic criteria for diagnosing AD in 1991 in an effort to facilitate sharing of case information reliably across multiple centers (Mirra et al., 1991). NSP were used as the primary lesion in the belief that this type of 'mature' plaque had a greater effect, compared to 'benign' DSP, in disrupting neuronal pathways and causing dementia. An age-adjusted NSP score was generated based on the maximum number of NSP detected in any of the four neocortical lobes. The number of tangles was also scored semi-quantitatively, yet this assessment did not enter into the final diagnosis. Senile plaque (SP) and neurofibrillary tangle (NFT) lesion scoring was facilitated by reference to cartoons showing 2, 6, and 28 NSP or NFT as equivalent to 'mild', 'moderate', and 'severe'. This implied the build-up of both SP and NFT was curvilinear and not linear with time. This function was not stipulated in the 1991 paper nor was it fitted to any experimental data.

Table 3.2 NIA-Khachaturian 1985 age-adjusted criteria for diagnosing Alzheimer's disease

'Minimum microscopic criteria' (per single 1 sq mm field neocortex)	
Below 50 years	2–5 SP *and* NFT
50 to 65 years	≥ 8 SP + some NFT
66 to 75 years	≥10 SP + some NFT
Over 75 years	≥15 SP ± some NFT

(Khachaturian, 1985)

The NIA-Reagan Institute criteria for diagnosing AD

The CERAD neuritic SP scoring system was incorporated into the 1997 NIA–Reagan Institute criteria and thus survives. Thus, an NSP score is first obtained and then a Braak NFP score is assigned to arrive at a probability score for that brain having pathologic AD as 'low', 'moderate' (or intermediate), or 'high'.

NIA–Reagan Institute criteria were developed to assess pathologic lesions including senile plaques and neurofibrillary tangles in demented brains only. Thus, the criteria *by definition* are not suitable to assess preclinical pathologic AD. By this system most CDR 0.5 subjects who have definite pathologic criteria by modified Khachaturian criteria have 'low probability' AD by NIA–Reagan Institute pathologic criteria. Research performed at the author's ADRC convincingly demonstrates that abundant neocortical DSP with some NSP are the best marker for the onset of very early AD (Morris & Price, 2001). For this reason, the author continues to stress the overall utility of Washington University ADRC modified Khachaturian criteria for the full spectrum of AD pathology ranging from none (CDR 0) to preclinical disease and later stages of very mild (CDR 0.5), mild (CDR 1), moderately severe (CDR 2), and severe (CDR 3) clinical AD. The original and Washington University modified Khachaturian NIA consensus diagnostic criteria quantify both DSP and NSP. In doing so, these criteria do acknowledge that some neocortical NFTs are intrinsic to AD pathogenesis. Of interest, the cut-points defined for the Washington University ADRC modified Khachaturian criteria (McKeel *et al.*, 2004) fall precisely in the plaque density range designated in the original publication (Khachaturian, 1985) (*Box 3.1*).

Box 3.1 Neuropathologic core features of dementing disorders

Core criteria for diagnosing AD
- Very mild, preclinical: neocortical widespread diffuse SP, rare NFT (Braak I–III)
- Mild to severe: increasing cortical NSP, NFT, NT (Braak III–VI)

Core criteria for diagnosing DLB
- DLB brainstem (brainstem > 5/section; limbic, cortical CLB <5/section)
- DLB limbic (limbic > CLB 5/section; cortical <5/section, most brainstem >5)
- DLB neocortical (cortex CLB >5/section)

Core criteria for diagnosing FTD
- Frontal and/or temporal lobar atrophy
- Severe lobar neuronal loss
- Severe lobar gliosis (with neuron loss)
- Superficial cortical microvacuolation
- Tau+ neuronal and glial inclusions in gray matter and white matter, variable (DLDH none)

Core criteria for diagnosing VaD
- Three or more infarcts c/w dementia duration (disregard acute)
- Presence of recognized ischemic pathology: arterio/atherosclerosis, CAA, cortical laminar necrosis, chronic hemorrhages, recurrent strokes
- Elevated Hachinski score >7

AD: Alzheimer's disease; CAA: cerebral amyloid angiopathy; CLB: cortical Lewy body; DLB: dementia with Lewy body; DLDH: dementia lacking distinctive histopathology; FTD: frontotemporal dementia; NFT: neurofibrillary tangle; NSP: neuritic senile plaque; NT: neuropil thread; VaD: vascular dementia

Histologic dyes and IHC, antibody-based methods

Conventional dye methods

Methods described here are generally useful for assessing the full spectrum of neurodegenerative disorders in adults: H&E, Nissl methods for neurons, thioflavine S, Congo red, luxol fast blue (LFB)- PAS, modified Bielschowsky silver (20% silver nitrate), Hedreen–Bielschowsky silver (4% cupric nitrate, 4% silver nitrate), and Gallyas silver.

Hematoxylin and eosin

This venerable histopathologic general screening stain has many 'flavors'. The use of eosin preparations with too much red obscure many diagnostic features that define neurodegenerative disorders (SP, Lewy bodies). Eosin solutions containing phloxine have proven to be optimal in the author's hands. Hematoxylin is a complex dye mixture that is 'blued' by running tap water. A robust intense blue that allows the full color range of eosin to be appreciated is the desired staining effect.

Recognition of pathognomonic inclusions that define dementing disorders using H&E may be difficult except in the case of classical haloed Lewy bodies (refer to Chapter 6). The H&E protocol the author uses (see Appendix) also gives excellent discrimination for hippocampal granulo-vacuoles and Hirano bodies, cortical Lewy bodies, a subset of SPs, and intraneuronal and extracellular NFTs. This method is highly recommended to diagnose dementing disorders and is illustrated throughout this book. Other dye stains are useful in defining human normal and pathologic neuroanatomy as shown (**3.4**).

3.4 A: Ballooned neurons filled with PAS-positive diastase-resistant granular secondary lysosomes in a case of adult ceroid lipofuscinosis (×40 objective). **B**: Cortical Lewy body and associated neurites labeled by alpha synuclein antibody (×40 objective). **C**: Apple-green birefringence of a beta-amyloid-containing cerebral artery that has been stained with Congo red and is viewed with cross polarizing filters (×10 objective). **D**: Fluorescently tagged antibody to PHF tau (white boutons) that differ from the argyrophilic swollen neurites of a neuritic senile plaque that has been stained by the de Olmos silver method (×60 objective oil immersion).

Nissl staining for neurons

Classical neuroanatomists still make frequent use of relatively thick (40–50 μm) frozen sections of cryoprotected aldehyde-fixed human brains for assessing neuronal populations. Toluidine blue and cresyl echt violet are the dyes of choice. The crucial factor of a successful Nissl protocol is to obtain a crystal clear background. For example, in neuronal stereology, it is critical to be able to see nuclear membranes and nucleoli clearly. The protocol used at the Washington University ADRC was developed in the laboratory of Dr Joseph L Price to map AD lesions on large (50 μm) frozen brain sections (Morris & Price, 2001).

Thioflavine S

Thioflavines are a family of fluorescent dyes (thioflavine S and T are most often used in pathology laboratories) that are economical and effective in visualizing AD lesions such as SP, NFT, and cerebral amyloid angiopathy (CAA), as an adjunct to H&E screening (**3.5**) (Delacourte *et al.*, 1987; Vickers *et al.*, 2003). Lesions are moderately to intensely green-yellow fluorescent against a pale background of neuropil. The specific lesions of AD are easily distinguished from the orange autofluorescence of lipofuscin that accumulates in many human neurons as part of the normal aging process (Porta, 2002).

Thioflavine S is also widely used to assess 'fibrillar' b-amyloid plaques in transgenic amyloid precursor protein (APP) mice (Games *et al.*, 1991; Brendza *et al.*, 2003). The results of plaque staining in transgenic mice that overexpress a-beta protein differ in some important respects from human AD amyloid deposits. For example, most of the diffuse neocortical amyloid 'plaques' in PDAPP mice are

3.5 Thioflavine S stained 6 μm paraffin sections viewed by epifluoresence with a fluorescein type filter. **A**: Fluorescent senile plaques (SP), neurofibrillary tangles (NFT), and neuronal cytoplasmic lipofuscin (arrow) in the cortex of an advanced Alzheimer patient (×20 objective). **B**: Beta-amyloid-containing cerebral capillaries, some with spike-like projections (dyshoria), in longitudinal and cross-sectional views (×40 objective). **C**: Leptomeningeal arteries, two of which have double lumens that are caused by mural deposition of beta-amyloid (×10 objective). **D**: Dyshoric reaction of a small cerebral artery with segmental involvement of the wall by beta-amyloid (×10 objective).

thioflavine S-negative in contrast to the thioflavine S-*positive* earliest diffuse beta-amyloid plaques that accumulate in Down's (trisomy 21) syndrome brains from affected individuals who die in their teens and 20s (**3.6**). A likely explanation is that thioflavine S-negative amyloid deposits conform to human 'preamyloid plaques'. These early plaque forms were defined by Tagliavini *et al.* (1988) as plaques that immunolabel with a-beta antibodies but are negative using silver methods, Congo red and thioflavine S.

Thioflavine S also dramatically highlights neuronal lipopigment in the adult form of Kuf's ceroid lipofuscinosis storage disease (**3.7**) (Josephson *et al.*, 2001). Affected neurons are ballooned and the cytoplasm is filled with intensely fluorescent granular deposits. Lewy bodies are generally only faintly positive with thioflavine stains and Lewy neurites are not stained (see Chapter 7). The tauopathy lesions of FTD cases (see Chapter 8), unlike AD tangles, are mostly silver-, Congo red- (see below), and thioflavine S-negative. Straight filament tangles in PSP are thioflavine S-negative and Bielschowsky silver-positive.

Congo red

Congo red (CR) is the classic dye staining 'gold standard' method for histologically defining the entire family of amyloidoses. The common feature of all amyloids, systemic and localized, is the presence of a high content of beta-pleated sheet substructure. CR dye molecules intercalate into molecular 'slots' formed by the beta-pleated sheets and thereby define a true amyloid protein as being CR-positive and exhibiting apple-green birefringence under polarized illumination. SP cores, NFTs and CAA (see **3.4C**) all exhibit this property.

Luxol fast blue-periodic acid Schiff

LFB-PAS has become the favorite stain for assessing brain myelin integrity in neuropathology laboratories around the world. The term 'Klüver–Barrera stain' (Akiguchi *et al.*, 2004) is synonymous. Intact myelin is stained an intense aqua blue color in contrast to demyelinated areas which are a paler blue color (**3.8**). The PAS component of LFB-PAS is useful for defining corpora amylacea, a subset

3.6 Multiple fluorescent diffuse Alzheimer beta amyloid plaques (arrows) are revealed by the thioflavine S technique in the cerebral cortex of a 24-year-old nondemented (CDR 0) woman who had trisomy 21 Down's syndrome. No tau-immunoreactive pathology was evident anywhere in this brain, and the plaques lacked tau-positive dystrophic neurites. The plaques also stained with the Hedreen–Bielschowsky method (×10 objective).

3.7 Thioflavine S method clearly reveals widespread swollen neocortical neurons which show massive pathologic accumulation of cytoplasmic lipopigment granules. Adult ceroid lipofuscinosis (Kuf's disease) patient (×40 objective, epifluorescent illumination).

of AD senile plaques, lipofuscin and ceroid granules, vascular basement membranes, gitter cell macrophage granules, and coarse granules in perivascular cells (pericytes, resting microglia).

Modified Bielshowsky silver stains

Dr Alois Alzheimer used Dr Bielschowsky's 1896 axonal silver method for defining senile plaques and neurofibrillary in the first reported case of AD in 1907. The diagnostic usefulness of this stain for diagnosing AD and displaying axons is thus well established and continuing. The Washington University ADRC Neuropathology Core laboratory has developed two variations that are useful for assessing NFTs and NSPs (see modified Bielschowsky silver protocol in the Appendix; 20% silver nitrate) and for total diffuse and neuritic SP using computer image analysis (Hibbard *et al.*, 1994; Cullen *et al.*, 1996) (see Hedreen–Bielschowsky silver in the Appendix; 4% cupric nitrate–4% silver nitrate). The different results obtained with the two methods are shown in figure **3.9**.

A great deal has been written about the relative merits of traditional silver methods versus IHC antibody-based methods for assessing AD plaques and tangles. Experience with parallel use of both methods over 15 years at the author's ADRC indicates that both silver and IHC methods are complementary. Each type of methodology has its own merits and pitfalls. It is often stated that silver methods are 'unreliable' or 'capricious' (and therefore not very useful in a modern setting). Yet silver methods work on archival brains stored for decades in formalin. Silver staining quality can be optimized by using fresh reagents and scrupulously clean acid-washed glassware. Under such conditions, these two silver methods are as reliable as antibody-based methods that have their own limitations. Figure **3.10** illustrates silver and IHC results in staining AD brain sections to assess SP and NFT. Washington University ADRC unpublished data (DW McKeel, Jr, K Powlishta, and NS Havlioglu) demonstrate both methods produce statistically comparable SP density counts, whereas tau immunostaining demonstrates elevated tangle counts due to pretangles that are not visualized with silver methods.

3.8 Kluver–Barrera luxol fast blue-periodic acid Schiff stain is a mainstay for examining myelin pathology. Normal myelin (**A**) stains uniformly blue. The nuclei belong to white matter oligodendrocytes and astrocytes (larger and clearer nuclei). In contrast, damaged myelin in **B** exhibits less intense nonuniform blue staining. Myelin has a circular, segmented pattern that differs from the more linear pattern of normal myelin sheaths. Such pathologically altered myelin would appear to be 'pale' in H&E screening sections (×20 objective).

While monoclonal antibodies (mabs) are said to be '100% specific' for their antigen, practical experience indicates that multiple dissimilar epitopes are recognized by individual mabs. This raises the real possibility that some mabs are not derived from a true single cell hybridoma clone. Alternatively, the immunizing antigen may not be pure. Many mabs recognize tissue sections epitopes that are sensitive to chemical fixatives (such as 10% commercial formalin), heat, or exposure to organic solvents (ethanol, toluene, xylene) during tissue processing and embedding in paraffin wax prior to sectioning on a microtome. Thus, the final histologic result achieved using IHC methods may depend not only on antibody purity and specificity, but also on the chemical fixation and tissue processing protocols that were used.

3.9 A: Less intense staining of Alzheimer senile plaques (SP) by the modified Bielschowsky (mBT; 20% silver nitrate) method, compared to the Hedreen–Bielschowsky (hmBP; 4% cupric nitrate–4% silver nitrate) method (**B**). Neurofibrillary tangles and argyrophilic plaque neurites are best viewed with mBT, while hmBP stained diffuse and neuritic SP are darker and provide enhanced contrast for robust quantitation and detection by image analysis. (Adjacent 6 μm paraffin section, ×10 objective.)

3.10 Alzheimer senile plaque detection is often less robust comparing the traditional and widely used modified Bielschowsky silver method (**A**) with the more modern beta-amyloid immunohistochemical technique employing a brown diaminobenzidine substrate (**B**) on near-serial 6 μm paraffin sections (×10 objective).

There are numerous examples from the AD field where the immunogen was 'purified tangles', yet some resulting antibodies when applied to AD brain tissue labeled SPs instead of NFTs (Masters *et al.*, 1985; Schmidt *et al.*, 1997)! Another example where disparate staining results can arise during immunostaining is the antibody Alz-50 (Ksiezak-Reding *et al.*, 1988) directed near the N-terminus of tau. The 441 amino acid tau molecule becomes truncated by proteolysis as AD progresses. Hippocampal CA1, entorhinal cortex and cortical areas of neuron loss and intense tangle formation ultimately result in conversion of some intraneuronal NFTs to the extracellular form (Augustinack *et al.*, 2001; Vickers *et al.*, 2003). Alz-50 IHC may show reduced labeling of tangles as a result. Such 'immunonegative' tangles, which nevertheless exist but can't be 'seen' by particular antibodies, may produce spuriously low quantitative counts when assessed by image analysis or stereologic techniques, for example.

None of the many steps in IHC staining methods have yet been standardized. This applies to type and times of fixation, embedding parameters including the effects of use of different 'paraffin' preparations that differ in composition (many contain 'plasticizers' and proprietary [unnamed] components, for example), application of antigen 'rescue' or 'unmasking' techniques, and the use of standardized antibodies or working dilutions, buffers, and substrates to name but some of the nonstandardized steps common to all immunostaining procedures. A working committee of European Neuropathologists is working on standardizing neuropathologic IHC methodology (Dennis Dickson, AANP 6/23/04, comment to Li *et al.*, 2004 [agonal factors on human CNS biochemistry]).

Gallyas silver method

This now widely used silver method uses a different underlying principle than the Bielschowsky methods. The Washington University ADRC has adapted the Gallyas method of Braak and Braak (1991b) to 6 μm paraffin sections in order to demonstrate a range of pathologic lesions. The Gallyas method is especially useful for visualizing extracellular and neuronal tangles, argyrophilic grain pathology, tau-positive neuritic changes, and glioneuronal inclusions in FTD tauopathic disorders, in displaying glial cell inclusions (GCI) to define multiple system atrophy (MSA) cases, and as another method to see CAA in paraffin sections (**3.11**). This list of Gallyas silver-positive lesions is not meant to be exhaustive.

IHC methods

Some caveats that have been expressed about interpreting results of IHC methodology in diagnosing dementing disorders have been covered in the preceding section. These limitations should be considered when choosing a particular antibody to use for diagnostic purposes. Unlike many clinical laboratory procedures, IHC methods with rare exceptions (ERB and HER-1 for breast cancer, for example) have not been subject to regulation or accreditation programs. Hospital-based diagnostic pathology laboratories are stringently regulated in the US; however, many IHC techniques are carried out in unregulated research laboratories.

The following IHC methods identify the major diagnostic cellular features for five major groups of neurodegenerative disorders: (1) AD – a-beta and tau; (2) Lewy disorders including MSA with GCI – alpha-synucleinopathies; (3) FTD disorders – tau, ubiquitin; (4) MND – alpha-synuclein, tau, ubiquitin; (5) vascular disease, cerebral angiopathy – a-beta amyloid; (6) disorders with gliosis – glial fibrillary acidic protein (GFAP); and (7) cerebral synapses – synaptophysin. *Box 3.2* describes the IHC markers for neurodegenerative diseases.

Beta amyloid (a-beta) IHC

Liberation of a 4 kd protein from insoluble brain amyloid fibrils was due to the use of formic acid (Klunk *et al.*, 1994). Selkoe *et al.* (1986) soon showed that '4 kd peptide' was the principle component of AD plaques. 4 kd was equivalent to the 40–43 amino acid beta amyloid protein discovered by Glenner and Wong (1984). A number of well characterized mabs directed at full length, 1–40 and 1–42 a-beta protein are now commercially available for use on paraffin sections of formalin fixed (PSFF) brains.

4G8 is a widely used mab that robustly immunostains full length a-beta in PSFF (Kraszpulski *et al.*, 1998). The 6F/3D a-beta clone also produced similar results. 'End specific' mabs that selectively recognized a-beta 1–40 and a-beta 1–42 in PSFF are also available from multiple commercial sources. Representative results using 10D5 (a gift of Dale Schenk at Elan Pharmaceuticals) and 4G8 a-beta mabs on normal and AD brains are shown in **3.12**.

3.11 A–D: Gallyas silver method applied to 6 μm paraffin human brain sections.
A: Demonstration of three major Alzheimer lesions: neuritic senile plaques (arrow), neurofibrillary tangles (short arrow), and neuropil threads (arrowhead) (×20 objective).
B: Two leptomeningeal microaneurysms (Gallyas-negative) surrounded by Gallyas-positive beta amyloid laden arteries (×10 objective).

C: Defining glial cell inclusions (GCI) in a case of multiple system atrophy (×40 objective). GCI are also labeled with alpha-synuclein antibodies (not shown here).
D: Argyrophilic grains of Braak in the entorhinal cortex of a patient with argyrophilic grain disease (×20 objective).

Box 3.2 Selected immunohistochemical markers for common lesions in neurodegenerative disease brains

- IL1-A (interleukin-1 alpha), LN-3 for activated microglia
- GFAP (glial fibrillary acidic protein) for normal and gliotic astrocytes
- Synaptophysin, synapsin, SNAP-25, alpha-synuclein for synapses
- Neuronal markers: Neu-N, ChAT (choline acetyltransferase) for cholinergic neurons, DBH (dopamine beta-hydroxylase) for dopaminergic neurons, TH (tyrosine hydroxylase) for noradrenergic neurons; Note: NSE (neuron specific enolase) is not entirely specific for neurons
- Dendritic spine markers: drebrin (Shim & Lubec, 2002)
- Myelin markers: MBP (myelin basic protein), ubiquitin (granular degeneration of aging)
- Alpha-synuclein for Lewy body and neurite pathology, GCI (glial cell inclusions) in multiple system atrophy, corpora amylacea
- Beta amyloid: Alzheimer senile plaques, cerebral amyloid angiopathy
- Hyperphosphorylated tau for Alzheimer neurofibrillary tangles and neuropil threads, Pick body inclusions, astrocytic plaques in corticobasal ganglionic degeneration, tufted astrocytes in progressive supranuclear palsy, argyrophilic grains of Braak in argyrophilic grain disease, and distinctive glial and neuronal inclusions in various tauopathies
- Alpha-internexin and neurofilament subunits for pathological neurofilament inclusions
- Ubiquitin for corpora amylacea, Lewy bodies and neurites, dentate fascia inclusions in frontotemporal dementia with motor neuron diseases, and dementia lacking distinctive histopathology
- Prion antibodies for transmissible spongiform encephalopathies (spontaneous and variant Creutzfeldt–Jakob disease), bovine spongiform encephalopathy, fatal familial insomnia, Gerstmann–Sträussler–Scheinker disease

3.12 Near-serial neocortical sections from an Alzheimer case reveal differences in beta-amyloid labeling by specific monoclonal antibody reagents using the brown diaminobenzamidine (DAB) substrate (**A**; 10D5, a gift from Athena/Elan and Dale Schenk) compared to red alkaline phosphatase (**B**; 4G8). Often the two substrates and antibodies provide comparable a-beta immunostaining results. 4G8 'sees' granular peri-Purkinje neuronal cerebellar deposits that are absent using 10D5 (×10 objective).

Tau IHC

Peter Davies and colleagues (Ksiezak-Reding *et al.*, 1988; Rye *et al.*, 1993) described an antibody (Alz-50) directed to the A68 antigen that was elevated in AD brains. Later, A68 was found (probably) to be a form of altered tau protein. Antibodies to certain hyperphosphorylated forms of tau protein that were specific for paired helical filament (PHF) component in AD neurofibrillary lesions were shown not to stain normal brain tau (Rye *et al.*, 1993). Today, 'PHFtau' antibodies directed to known phosphorylated sites on tau are widely used to visualize AD tangles, neuropil threads (NTs), and plaques, dystrophic neurites in AD brains, tau lesions in FTD tauopathies, and tangles that occur, for example, in PSP, postencephalitic parkinsonism, boxers' brains, and entorhinal cortex in normal aging.

The monoclonal antibody PHF-1 labels phosphorylated serines at positions 396 and 404 of tau (Greenberg *et al.*, 1992). This mab robustly immunostains PHFtau but not normal tau in paraffin sections of formalin fixed mammalian brain tissue. Mab AT8 produces very similar results (Kitamura *et al.*, 2005) (**3.13**). It, too, is directed at specific phosphorylation sites at positions serine 202 and threonine 205 of the tau molecule.

Combined IHC for a-beta and tau

At the author's ADRC a dual IHC method is used that combines a-beta 4G8 mab IHC with either PHF-1 or AT8 mab IHC. As shown in figure **3.14**, use of an alkaline phosphatase red substrate for a-beta and a blue-black substrate for PHFtau provides striking delineation of tau-positive neuritic plaques and tau-negative diffuse and preamyloid plaques simultaneously with a-beta immunoreactivity. At the same time, tau-positive NFTs and NTs display the full range of AD neurofibrillary pathology.

Alpha synuclein IHC

A major breakthrough in understanding the pathogenesis of Lewy body disorders (PD, DLB) was the recognition that the presynaptic protein alpha-synuclein became translocated in PD and DLB to form insoluble aggregates in the cytoplasm (classic and cortical Lewy bodies) as well as 'Lewy neurites' (LNs). LNs are akin to tau-positive NTs in AD. In the so-called CA2/3 sector of the hippocampus, which studies indicate often occupies the CA2/1 junctional area, cases of combined AD and PD/DLB may show florid accumulation of PHFtau and alpha-synuclein-positive immunoreactive neurites (**3.15**). It has not been well

3.13 An example of staining patterns of two among many robust hyperphosphorylated tau antibodies that are available to label cytoskeletal abnormalities in neurodegenerative disorders. **A**: Robust PHF-1 (a generous gift of Dr Peter Davies) immunostaining of hippocampal CA1 pathologic tangles and neuropil threads in advanced AD (×10). **B**: Equally robust labeling of a dense meshwork of neuropil threads, senile plaques, and neurofibrillary tangles by commercial tau antibody AT8 in the cerebral cortex of another advanced AD patient (×10 objective hematoxylin counterstain with DAB brown substrate). (Compare to **3.11**.)

3.14 Combining a-beta (antibody 4G8 or 10D5, red alkaline phosphate substrate) with tau (antibodies PHF- or AT8, true blue substrate) has proven very useful to discriminate conclusively tau-negative (red only, preamyloid and diffuse) and tau-positive (red with black, neuritic) senile plaques (one is shown at 3 o'clock), while simultaneously labeling black neurofibrillary tangles (at 9 o'clock position), neuropil threads (shown) and vascular beta amyloid (not illustrated) (×20 objective, 6 µm paraffin brain section).

3.15 Antibody to the presynaptic protein alpha-synuclein (Zymed LB-509 monoclonal antibody shown here) is the current method of choice for demonstrating Lewy pathology in dementia with Lewy bodies. A cortical Lewy body, a type of neuronal cytoplasmic inclusion, is shown at upper left, while a huge Lewy 'mega-neurite' is shown at lower right. Finer linear Lewy neurites are scattered through the field. Round punctate tiny objects are antibody labeled individual synapses (×40 objective).

established whether or not individual neuritic processes are co-labeled by both antibodies or whether co-mingled tau- and alpha synuclein-positive neuritic elements are observed.

Ubiquitin IHC

Proteins destined for cellular elimination are targeted to the 26S cytoplasmic proteosome by being 'tagged' by ubiquitin. There is additional recent evidence that alpha-synuclein and ubiquitin are both integral components of Lewy bodies (Snyder and Wolozin, 2004). Ubiquitin labels Lewy bodies, corpora amylacea (CA), some AD plaque and neuropil neurites, subsets of NFTs in AD brains, and white matter 'granular degeneration', a near universal accompaniment of human aging (**3.16**) (also see Chapter 4) (Wang *et al.*, 2004). Many polyclonal and monoclonal antibodies to

ubiquitin are commercially available. The author uses a polyclonal antibody from East Acres to achieve robust staining using PSFF. More recently, a mouse monoclonal antiubiquitin antibody has proven to be even more sensitive for detecting cytoplasmic and nuclear inclusions in cases of FTD–MND (**3.16**).

GFAP IHC

GFAP is the main component of one class of intermediate filament proteins that are found in astrocytic glial cells (Roelofs *et al.*, 2005). Pathologists use GFAP IHC to define 'gliosis'. This term refers to abnormal hypertrophy and hyperplasia of astrocytes in various pathologic disorders that range from normal aging, to brain infarction, to areas of neuron loss in AD and FTD (**3.17**).

3.16 A–F: East Acres polyclonal ubiquitin antiserum labeling. **A**: Strongly immunolabeled corpora amylacea (×20 objective). **B**: Rounded profiles, probably cross-sectioned dendrites, of unknown diagnostic significance, in the subiculum (×40 objective). **C**: Ubiquinated inclusions in dentate fascia neurons (×40 objective). **D**: Irregular curly ubiquinated neurites in neocortex of a frontotemporal dementia case (×40 objective). **E**: Strong ubiquitin labeling of neuritic plaque neurites in hippocampal area CA4 of an Alzheimer patient (×20 objective). **F**: Aging related, ubiquitin-positive, granular degeneration of the white matter (×40 objective). The additional uses of ubiquitin for revealing Lewy pathology are described in Chapter 7.

Synaptophysin IHC

Human brain synapses contain multiple marker proteins (Lippa *et al.*, 1992) that may be used to identify them in biochemical assays (dot and Western blotting) as well as by IHC on tissue sections (**3.18**) (Reddy *et al.*, 2005). Synapse protein quantification may be successfully achieved using optical density measurements of the IHC reaction product (Lippa *et al.*, 1992) or by counting the total number of synapses in a brain reference volume using unbiased stereology at the light (Calhoun *et al.*, 1996; DW McKeel, Jr and NS Havlioglu, unpublished data on 20 subjects CDR 0–3) or the ultrastructural (electron microscopic) level (DeKosky *et al.*, 1996). In the author's experience, excellent robust synaptophysin IHC results may be obtained on formalin-fixed paraffin-embedded (FFPE) brain sections up to 48 hours postmortem. A minority of brains (~20%) for unknown reasons fail to stain robustly enough with synaptophysin antibodies to perform stereologic analysis (NS Havlioglu and DW McKeel, Jr, unpublished data).

Synaptophysin immunoreactivity was decreased significantly in both AD prefrontal cortex (Masliah *et al.*, 2001) and in terminal fields of the perforant pathway located in the molecular layer of the hippocampal dentate fascia (Morys *et al.*, 1994; NS Havlioglu and DW McKeel, Jr, unpublished data) in brains from patients with very mild (CDR 0.5) AD. The latter study revealed that synaptophysin immunoreactivity declined throughout the CDR with a Pearson correlation between last CDR and total synapse number in the entire left hippocampus of $r = 0.85$. Unbiased sampling and stereology methodology thus produced the highest positive correlation observed between AD dementia severity (CDR assessment) and an established neuropathology biomarker of disease.

3.17 Astrocytic hypertrophy and hyperplasia, gliosis, is a fundamental pathologic process in many neuro-degenerative disorders. Antibodies to glial fibrillary acid protein, a class of astrocytic intermediate filaments, is extensively used to reveal pathologic gliosis in human neuropathology. (DAB substrate, 6 μm paraffin section, ×20 objective.)

3.18 Antibodies to synaptophysin (DAB brown substrate) are often used to label and quantify synapses as shown here in the hippocampal dentate fascia. Clusters and individual synapses may be seen within the superimposed frame of the optical disector (asterisk: out of frame in focus synapse, arrow: out of frame, out of focus plane synapse), when viewed at ×3200 final magnification with the PC-based Stereologer™ image analysis and stereology system. The cellular nuclei have been counterstained with hematoxylin (×100 oil immersion). (DG, dentate gyrus; SGL supragranular layer.)

Newer diagnostic methods for dementing disorders

Newer diagnostic methods have been developed that provide major insights into key mechanisms of disease that determine cognitive impairment and dementia across the spectrum of related disorders. Some of them are described in the following sections.

Tissue microarrays

Tissue microarrays (Sjobeck *et al.*, 2003; Simon *et al.*, 2005), small cores of paraffin embedded formalin-fixed archival brain tissue, are re-embedded in new paraffin blocks in a 'row and column matrix' of similar sized tissue cores on a regular 1 × 3 inch glass slide (**3.19**). Depending on the diameter of each core (usually 0.6–3 mm), densities as high as 50–100 cores per slide can be constructed. In this manner, new antibodies can be screened, or series of similar cases can be assessed for individual case differences to, for example, a single standard antibody (**3.20**).

Laser capture tissue microdissection and biochemical microanalysis

Laser and microscope-based instrumentation is now available so that single cells or lesions, such as individual Alzheimer SPs, may be isolated with the laser from a fixed histologic section, affixed onto film, and carried through staining solutions or pooled for biochemical microanalysis. Nucleic acid concentrations including mRNA may be determined. This technology is finding wide application in neurodegenerative disease research (Hyman *et al.*, 2005; Standaert, 2005).

Multiphoton brain tissue microscopy

Single, dual, triple, or even four-photon microscopic methods are available to visualize structures located several hundred microns below the brain surface in living animals (Denk *et al.*, 1994). Typical applications involve introduction of tracers directly onto the brain surface or intravenously. For example, a brain soluble marker, such as the fluorescent dye thioflavine S, can gain entry into the

3.19 Six cerebral cortex cores of a neurodegenerative disorders tissue microarray are shown after staining with anti-4G8 (amyloid beta) and AT8 tau antibody dual label immunohistochemistry (please refer to **3.14**). Blank microarray slide courtesy of Dr Irina Alafuzoff as part of a NACC methodological collaborative study between European and US Alzheimer Disease Center neuropathology laboratories. Note absence of both a-beta and tau labeling in the section at far upper right, and variable amounts of amyloid (red) and tau (black) among the other brain tissue cores (×1 objective). (Compare with figure **3.20**.)

3.20 One of the dual immunolabeled tissue cores from **3.19** is shown at higher magnification to display quality of staining. The result is in every way comparable to larger sections that have been individually processed and stained. Neuritic senile plaques, neurofibrillary tangles, neuropil threads, and parenchymal vascular amyloid deposition are clearly revealed in the small tissue core sample (×10 objective). (Compare with figure **3.19**.)

brain through a thin or open window in the skull (D'Amore *et al.*, 2003). The dye infiltrates the brain and rapidly binds to senile plaques which fluoresce. By carefully marking the 3-dimensional spatial location of a particular plaque, serial observations are possible over time as to whether the plaque grows in size, maintains a stable size, or diminishes in size and disappears. Examples of all three types have been observed in mouse models of AD (Christie *et al.*, 2001).

Determination of beta-amyloid load or burden

Image analysis and stereologic methods may be used to quantify the fractional area occupied by beta-amyloid protein in histologic slides of brain neocortex. This approach obviates the tedious task of counting thousands of individual Alzheimer senile plaques in a single tissue section. This measure has been referred to as the 'amyloid burden' or the 'amyloid load' (Hyman *et al.*, 1993; Leverenz *et al.*, 1998) (**3.21**).

New combinatorial or hybrid methods to visualize AD lesions

Rapid advances in biomedical engineering, in the physical and chemical sciences, and in molecular biology, have led to powerful methods to gain insights into mechanisms of neurodegenerative diseases, including EM and stereology (Dunckley *et al.*, 2006), comparing IHC with quantitative AD marker biochemistry (Feany & Dickson, 1996; Jackson and Lowe, 1996), and multiphoton microscopy of fluorescent oxidation products that localize in senile plaques (McLellan *et al.*, 2003). The development of *in vivo* radiochemical probes that bind directly to senile plaques allowing them to be visualized in living patients by positive emission tomography (PET) promises to revolutionize AD diagnosis and treatment monitoring (Nordberg, 2004; Verhoeff *et al.*, 2004; Price *et al.*, 2005).

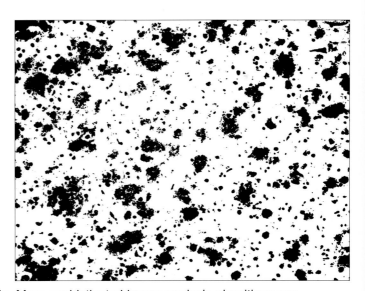

3.21 This color-converted TIFF black and white image of an Alzheimer cerebral cortex 6 μm thick section, which had been stained by an a-beta specific antibody and a link antibody with a red chromogen, was manually thresholded and converted to binary in Adobe *Photoshop CS*. The black senile plaque pixels (44418 pixels) represent 22.16% of the total image area (200720 pixels). The image was captured by an ISI Colorview II™ digital camera at 72 dpi in a 28K × 22K pixel image that then was resized to 6 inches wide by 4.4 inches high at 300 dpi for publication. The section was viewed with a ×10 microscope objective on a Nikon E-800 Eclipse research microscope in the Washington University ADRC Neuropathology Core Laboratory. The basic method is widely used to determine the fractional area ('burden' or 'load') occupied by beta-amyloid protein in the Alzheimer brain. More sophisticated image analysis algorithms are available to generate similar data (Hibbard *et al.*, 1994, 1995, 1997).

References

Akiguchi I, Tomimoto H, Wakita H, *et al.* (2004). Topographical and cytopathological lesion analysis of the white matter in Binswanger's disease brains. *Acta Neuropathol.* **107**:563–570.

Alzheimer A (1907). Über eine eignartiger Erkrankung der Hirnrinde (About a peculiar disease of the cerebral cortex); English translation in *Alz. Dis. Ass. Dis.* **1**:7–8, 1987. *Allgemeine Zeitschrift fur Psychiatrie und Psychisch-Gerichtliche Medizin* **64**:146–148.

Augustinack JC, Schneider A, Mandelkow EM, *et al.* (2002). Specific tau phosphorylation sites correlate with severity of neuronal cytopathology in Alzheimer's disease. *Acta Neuropathol.* **103**:26–35.

Bellomo G, Santambrogio L, Fiacconi M, *et al.* (1991). Plasma profiles of adrenocorticotropic hormone, cortisol, growth hormone, and prolactin in patients with untreated Parkinson's disease. *J. Neurol.* **238**:19–22.

Berg L, McKeel DW, Jr., Miller JP, *et al.* (1998). Clinicopathologic studies in cognitively healthy aging and Alzheimer disease: relation of histologic markers to dementia severity, age, sex, and apolipoprotein E genotype. *Arch. Neurol.* **55**:326–335.

Bertram L, Tanzi RE (2004). The current status of Alzheimer's disease genetics: what do we tell the patients? [Review] [83 refs] *Pharmacol. Res.* **50**:385–396.

Blackwell AD, Sahakian BJ, Vesey R, *et al.* (2004). Detecting dementia: novel neuropsychological markers of preclinical Alzheimer's disease. *Dementia & Geriatric Cognitive Dis.* **17**:42–48.

Braak H, Braak E (1991a). The neuropathologic stageing of Alzheimer-related changes. *Acta Neuropathol* (Berlin) **82**:239–259.

Braak H, Braak E (1991b). Demonstration of amyloid deposits and neurofibrillary changes in whole brain sections. *Brain Pathol.* **1**:213–216.

Brendza RP, O'Brien C, Simmons K, *et al.* (2003). PDAPP YFP double transgenic mice: a tool to study amyloid-beta associated changes in axonal, dendritic, and synaptic structures. *J. Comp. Neurol.* **456**:375–383.

Calhoun ME, Jucker M, Martin LJ, *et al.* (1996). Comparative evaluation of synaptophysin-based methods for quantification of synapses. *J. Neurocytol.* **25**:821–828.

Christie RH, Bacskai BJ, Zipfel WR, *et al.* (2001). Growth arrest of individual senile plaques in a model of Alzheimer's disease observed by *in vivo* multiphoton microscopy. *J. Neurosci.* **21**:858–864.

Crystal H, Dickson D, Fuld P, *et al.* (1988). Clinico-pathologic studies in dementia. Nondemented subjects with pathologically confirmed Alzheimer's disease. *Neurology* **38**:1682–1687.

Cullen KM, Halliday GM, Cartwright H, *et al.* (1996). Improved selectivity and sensitivity in the visualization of neurofibrillary tangles, plaques and neuropil threads. *Neurodegeneration* **5**:177–187.

D'Amore JD, Kajdasz ST, McLellan ME, *et al.* (2003). *In vivo* multiphoton imaging of a transgenic mouse model of Alzheimer disease reveals marked thioflavine-S-associated alterations in neurite trajectories. *J. Neuropathol. Exp. Neurol.* **62**:137–145.

de Carvalho M (2001). Pathophysiological significance of fasciculations in the early diagnosis of ALS. *Amyotrophic Lateral Sclerosis & Other Motor Neuron Disorders* Suppl 1:S43–S46.

DeKosky ST, Scheff SW, Styren SD (1996). Structural correlates of cognition in dementia: quantification and assessment of synapse change. [Review] [32 refs] *Neurodegeneration* **5**:417–421.

Denk W, Delaney KR, Gelperin A, *et al.* (1994). Anatomical and functional imaging of neurons using 2-photon laser scanning microscopy. [Review] [35 refs] *J. Neurosci. Meth.* **54**:151–162.

Desai AK, Grossberg GT (2005). Diagnosis and treatment of Alzheimer's disease. *Neurology* **64**(12 Suppl 3):S34–S39.

Delacourte A, Defossez A, Persuy P, *et al.* (1987). Observation of morphological relationships between angiopathic blood vessels and degenerative neurites in Alzheimer's disease. *Virchows Archiv – A, Pathological Anatomy & Histopathology* **411**:199–204.

Dickson DW (2003). *Neurodegeneration: The Molecular Pathology of Dementia and Movement Disorders*. ISN Neuropath. Press, Basel.

Dunckley T, Beach TG, Ramsey K, *et al.* (2006). Gene expression correlates of neurofibrillary tangles in Alzheimer's disease. *Neurobiol. Aging* **27**:1359–1371.

Esiri MM, Hyman BT, Beyreuther K, *et al.* (1997). Ageing and dementia. In: *Greenfield's Neuropathology* (6th edn.). DI Graham, PL Lantos (eds.). Arnold, London, pp. 153–234.

Esiri MM, Lee V-MY, Trojanowski JQ (ed.) (2004). *The Neuropathology of Dementia*. Cambridge University Press, Cambridge.

Feany MB, Dickson DW (1996). Neurodegenerative disorders with extensive tau pathology: a comparative study and review. [Review] [93 refs] *Ann. Neurol.* **40**:139–148.

Flynn MD, Cundy TF, Watkins PJ (1988). Antepartum pituitary necrosis in diabetes mellitus. [Review] [10 refs] *Diabetic Med.* **5**:295–297.

Forman MS, Lee VM, Trojanowski JQ (2005a). Nosology of Parkinson's disease: looking for the way out of a quagmire. [Review] [26 refs] *Neuron* **47**:479–482.

Forman MS, Mackenzie IR, Markesbery WR, *et al.* (2005b). Novel ubiquitin brain pathology in frontotemporal dementia with inclusion body myopathy and Paget's disease. (abstract 12) Am. Assoc. Neuropathol. *J. Neuropathol. Exp. Neurol.* **64**:433.

Fowler MR, McKeel DW Jr (1979a). Human adenohypophyseal quantitative histochemical cell classification. I. Morphologic criteria and cell type distribution. *Arch. Pathol. Lab. Med.* **103**:613–620.

Fowler MR, McKeel DW Jr (1979b). Human adenohypophyseal quantitative histochemical cell classification. II. Evaluation of the effects of two fixatives and postmortem interval. *Arch. Pathol. Lab. Med.* **103**:621–623.

Games D, Adams D, Allesandrini R, *et al.* (1991). Alzheimer-type neuropathology in transgenic mice overexpressing V717F beta-amyloid precursor protein. *Nature* **349**:704–706.

Giannakopoulos P, Hof PR, Kovari E, *et al.* (1996). Distinct patterns of neuronal loss and Alzheimer's disease lesion distribution in elderly individuals older than 90 years. *J. Neuropathol. Exp. Neurol.* **55**:1210–1220.

Glenner GG, Wong CW (1984). Alzheimer's disease: initial report of the purification and characterization of a novel cerebrovascular amyloid protein. *Biochem. Biophys. Res. Comm.* **120**:885–890.

Goldman WP, Storandt M, Miller JP, *et al.* (2001). Mild cognitive impairment represents early-stage Alzheimer's disease. *Arch. Neurol.* **58**:397–405.

Greenberg SG, Davies P, Schein JD, *et al.* (1992). Hydrofluoric acid-treated tau PHF proteins display the same biochemical properties as normal tau. *J. Biol. Chem.* **267**:564–569.

Grundman M, Petersen RC, Ferris SH, *et al.* (2004). Alzheimer's Disease Cooperative Study. Mild cognitive impairment can be distinguished from Alzheimer disease and normal aging for clinical trials. *Arch. Neurol.* **61**:59–66.

Hibbard LS, McKeel DW Jr, Arnicar-Sulze TL, *et al.* (1994). Automated detection and morphological analysis of senile plaques in SDAT. *J. Neurosci. Meth.* **52**:175–189.

Hibbard LS, McKeel DW Jr (1995). Multiscale detection and analysis of senile plaques of Alzheimer's disease. *IEEE Transactions on Pattern Analysis and Machine Intelligence* **42**:1218–1225.

Hibbard LS, McKeel DW Jr (1997). Automated identification and quantitative morphometry of the senile plaques of Alzheimer's disease. *Analytical Quant. Cytol. Histol.* **19**:123–138.

Holton JL, Révész T, Crooks R, *et al.* (2001). Evidence for pathological involvement of the spinal cord in motor neuron disease-inclusion dementia. *Acta Neuropathol.* **103**:221–227.

Horvath E, Kovacs K, Scheithauer BW (1999). Pituitary hyperplasia. [Review] [60 refs] *Pituitary* **1**:169–179.

Hughes CP, Berg L, Danziger WL, *et al.* (1982). A new clinical scale for the staging of dementia. *Br. J. Psych.* **140**:566–572.

Hyman BT, Augustinack JC, Ingelsson M (2005). Transcriptional and conformational changes of the tau molecule in Alzheimer's disease. [Review] [73 refs] *Biochim. Biophys. Acta* **1739**:150–157.

Hyman BT, Marzloff K, Arriagada PV (1993). The lack of accumulation of senile plaques or amyloid burden in Alzheimer's disease suggests a dynamic balance between amyloid deposition and resolution. *J. Neuropathol. Exp. Neurol.* **52**:594–600.

Jackson M, Lowe J (1996). The new neuropathology of degenerative frontotemporal dementias. [Review] [38 refs] *Acta Neuropathol.* **91**:127–134.

Josephson SA, Schmidt RE, Millsap P, *et al.* (2001). Autosomal dominant Kufs' disease: a cause of early onset dementia. *J. Neurol. Sci.* **188**:51–60.

Kato S, Hirano A, Llena JF (1992). Immuno-histochemical, ultrastructural, and immunoelectron microscopic studies of spinal cord neurofibrillary tangles in progressive supranuclear palsy. *Neuropathol. Appl. Neurobiol.* **18**:531–538.

Kanda T, Tsukagoshi H, Oda M, *et al.* (1996). Changes of unmyelinated nerve fibers in sural nerve in amyotrophic lateral sclerosis, Parkinson's disease, and multiple system atrophy. *Acta Neuropathol.* **91**:145–154.

Katzman R, Terry R, De Teresa R, *et al.* (1988). Clinical, pathological, and neurochemical changes in dementia: a subgroup with preserved mental status and numerous neocortical plaques. *Ann. Neurol.* **23**:138–144.

Kingsbury AE, Foster OJ, Nisbet AP, *et al.* (1995). Tissue pH as an indicator of mRNA preservation in human postmortem brain. *Brain Res. Mol. Brain Res.* **28**:311–318.

Kirshner HS (2005). Mild cognitive impairment: to treat or not to treat. *Curr. Neurol. Neurosci. Rep.* **5**:455–457.

Kitamura T, Sugimori K, Sudo S, *et al.* (2005). Relationship between microtubule-binding repeats and morphology of neurofibrillary tangle in Alzheimer's disease. *Acta Neurol. Scand.* **112**:327–334.

Khachaturian ZS (1985). Diagnosis of Alzheimer's disease. *Arch. Neurol.* **42**:1097–1105.

Klunk WE, Xu CJ, Pettegrew JW (1994). NMR identification of the formic acid-modified residue in Alzheimer's amyloid protein. *J. Neurochem.* **62**:349–354.

Klüver and Barrera (1953). A method for the combined staining of cells and fibers in the central nervous system. *J. Neuropath. Exp. Neurol.* **12**:400–403.

Kraszpulski M, Soininen H, Riekkinen P Sr, *et al.* (1998). Pitfalls in the quantitative estimation of beta-amyloid immunoreactivity in human brain tissue. *Histochem. Cell Biol.* **110**:439–445.

Ksiezak-Reding H, Davies P, Yen SH (1988). Alz-50, a monoclonal antibody to Alzheimer's disease antigen, cross-reacts with tau proteins from bovine and normal human brain. *J. Biol. Chem.* **263**:7943–7947.

Leverenz JB, Raskind MA (1998). Early amyloid deposition in the medial temporal lobe of young Down syndrome patients: a regional quantitative analysis. *Exp. Neurol.* **150**:296–304.

Li JZ, Vawter MP, Walsh DM, *et al.* (2004). Systematic changes in gene expression in postmortem human brains associated with tissue pH and terminal medical conditions. *Human Mol. Genet.* **13**:609–616.

Lippa CF, Hamos JE, Pulaski-Salo D, *et al.* (1992). Alzheimer's disease and aging: effects on perforant pathway perikarya and synapses. *Neurobiol. Aging* **13**:405–411.

Lowe J (1998). Establishing a neuropathological diagnosis in degenerative dementias. *Brain Pathol.* **8**:403–406.

Luna L (1968). *Manual of Histologic Staining Methods of the AFIP* (3rd edn.) McGraw-Hill Book Co., New York, pp. 203–204.

Luna L (1968). Schiff Reagent for the PAS (periodic acid-Schiff) stain: 21b. In: *Manual of Histologic Staining Methods of the AFIP* (3rd edn.) McGraw-Hill Book Co., New York, p. 159.

Luna-Munoz J, Garcia-Sierra F, Falcon V, *et al.* (2005). Regional conformational change involving phosphorylation of tau protein at the Thr231, precedes the structural change detected by Alz-50 antibody in Alzheimer's disease. *J. Alz. Dis.* **8**:29–41.

Markesbery WR (1998). *Neuropathology of Dementing Disorders*. Edward Arnold (Publishers) Limited, London. ISBN 0-340-59037-8; EAN: 9780340590379, pp. 404.

Masliah E, Mallory M, Alford M, *et al.* (2001). Altered expression of synaptic proteins occurs early during progression of Alzheimer's disease. *Neurology* **56**:127–129.

Masters CL, Multhaup G, Simms G, *et al.* (1985). Neuronal origin of a cerebral amyloid: neurofibrillary tangles of Alzheimer's disease contain the same protein as the amyloid of plaque cores and blood vessels. *EMBO J.* **4**:2757–2763.

McKeel DW Jr, Ball MJ, Price JL, *et al.* (1993). Interlaboratory histopathologic assessment of Alzheimer neuropathology: different methodologies yield comparable diagnostic results. *Alz. Dis. Assoc. Dis.* **7**:136–151.

McKeel DW Jr, Price JL, Miller, JP, *et al.* (2004). Neuropathologic criteria for diagnosing Alzheimer disease in persons with pure dementia of Alzheimer type. *J. Neuropathol. Exp. Neurol.* **63**:1028–1037.

McLellan ME, Kajdasz ST, Hyman BT, *et al.* (2003). *In vivo* imaging of reactive oxygen species specifically associated with thioflavine S-positive amyloid plaques by multiphoton microscopy. *J. Neurosci.* **23**:2212–2217.

Mirra SS, Gearing M, McKeel DW Jr, *et al.* (1994) Interlaboratory comparison of neuropathologic assessments in Alzheimer's disease: a study of the Consortium to Establish a Registry for Alzheimer's disease (CERAD). *J. Neuropathol. Exp. Neurol.* **53**:303–315.

Mirra SS, Heyman A, McKeel D Jr, *et al.* (1991). The Consortium to Establish a Registry for Alzheimer's Disease (CERAD). Part II. Standardization of the neuropathologic assessment of Alzheimer's disease. *Neurology* **41**:479–486.

Morihara T, Kudo T, Ikura Y, *et al.* (1998). Increased tau protein level in postmortem cerebrospinal fluid. *Psych. Clin. Neurosci.* **52**:107–110.

Morris JC (1993). The Clinical Dementia Rating (CDR): current version and scoring rules.[see comment]. *Neurology* **43**:2412–2414.

Morris JC, Price JL (2001). Pathologic correlates of nondemented aging, mild cognitive impairment, and early-stage Alzheimer's disease. [Review] [110 refs] *J. Mol. Neurosci.* **17**:101–118.

Morris JC, Storandt M, McKeel DW Jr, *et al.* (1996). Cerebral amyloid deposition and diffuse plaques in 'normal' aging: evidence for presymptomatic and very mild Alzheimer's disease. *Neurology* **46**:707–719.

Morys J, Sadowski M, Barcikowska M, *et al.* (1994). The second layer neurones of the entorhinal cortex and the perforant path in physiological ageing and Alzheimer's disease. *Acta Neurobiol. Exp.* **54**:47–53.

National Institute on Aging, and Reagan Institute Working Group on Diagnostic Criteria for Neuropathological Assessment of Alzheimer's disease (1997). Working Group Consensus Recommendations for the postmortem diagnosis of Alzheimer's disease. *Neurobiol. Aging* **18**(4 Suppl): S1–S2.

Nordberg A (2004). PET imaging of amyloid in Alzheimer's disease. [Review] [80 refs] *Lancet Neurol.* **3**:519–527.

Petersen RC (2004). Mild cognitive impairment as a diagnostic entity. [Review] [50 refs] *J. Int. Med.* **256**:183–194.

Porta EA (2002). Pigments in aging: an overview. [Review] [50 refs] *Ann. N.Y. Acad. Sci.* **959**:57–65.

Price JC, Klunk WE, Lopresti BJ, *et al.* (2005). Kinetic modeling of amyloid binding in humans using PET imaging and Pittsburgh Compound-B. *J. Cereb. Blood Flow Metab.* **25**:1528–1547.

Rademakers R, Cruts M, van Broeckhoven C (2004). The role of tau (MAPT) in frontotemporal dementia and related tauopathies. [Review] [195 refs] *Human Mutation* **24**:277–295.

Reddy PH, Mani G, Park BS, *et al.* (2005). Differential loss of synaptic proteins in Alzheimer's disease: implications for synaptic dysfunction. *J. Alz. Dis.* **7**:103–117; discussion 173–180.

Roelofs RF, Fischer DF, Houtman SH, *et al.* (2005). Adult human subventricular, subgranular, and subpial zones contain astrocytes with a specialized intermediate filament cytoskeleton. *GLIA* **52**:289–300.

Rye DB, Leverenz J, Greenberg SG, *et al.* (1993). The distribution of Alz-50 immunoreactivity in the normal human brain. *Neuroscience* **56**:109–127.

Schmidt ML, Lee VM, Forman M, *et al.* (1997). Monoclonal antibodies to a 100-kD protein reveal abundant A beta-negative plaques throughout gray matter of Alzheimer's disease brains. *Am. J. Pathol.* **151**:69–80.

Selkoe DJ, Abraham CR, Podlisny MB, *et al.* (1986). Isolation of low-molecular weight proteins from amyloid plaque fibers in Alzheimer's disease. *J. Neurochem.* **46**:1820–1824.

Shim KS, Lubec G (2002). Drebrin, a dendritic spine protein, is manifold decreased in brains of patients with Alzheimer's disease and Down syndrome. *Neurosci. Lett.* **324**:209–212.

Simon R, Mirlacher M, Sauter G (2005). Tissue microarrays. *Meth. Molec. Med.* **114**:257–268.

Sjobeck M, Haglund M, Persson A, Sturesson K, Englund E (2003). Brain tissue microarrays in dementia research: white matter microvascular pathology in Alzheimer disease. *Neuropathology* **23**:290–295.

Snyder H, Wolozin B (2004). Pathological proteins in Parkinson's disease: focus on the proteasome. [Review] [179 refs] *J. Mol. Neurosci.* **24**:425–442.

Standaert DG (2005). Applications of laser capture microdissection in the study of neurodegenerative disease. [Review] [10 refs] *Arch. Neurol.* **62**:203–205.

Strozyk D, Blennow K, White LR, *et al.* (2003). CSF Abeta 42 levels correlate with amyloid-neuropathology in a population-based autopsy study. *Neurology* **60**:652–656.

Tagliavini F, Giaccone G, Frangione B, *et al.* (1988). Preamyloid deposits in the cerebral cortex of patients with Alzheimer's disease and nondemented individuals. *Neurosci. Lett.* **93**:191–196.

Troost D, Das PK, van den Oord JJ, *et al.* (1992). Immunohistological alterations in muscle of patients with amyotrophic lateral sclerosis: mononuclear cell phenotypes and expression of MHC products. *Clin. Neuropathol.* **11**:115–120.

Vattemi G, Engel WK, McFerrin J, *et al.* (2003). Cystatin C colocalizes with amyloid-beta and coimmunoprecipitates with amyloid-beta precursor protein in sporadic inclusion-body myositis muscles. *J. Neurochem.* **85**:1539–1546.

Verhoeff NP, Wilson AA, Takeshita S, *et al.* (2004). *In vivo* imaging of Alzheimer disease beta-amyloid with [11C]SB-13 PET. *Am. J. Ger. Psych.* **12**:584–595.

Vickers JC, Tan A, Dickson TC (2003). Direct determination of the proportion of intra- and extracellular neocortical neurofibrillary tangles in Alzheimer's disease. *Brain Res.* **971**:135–137.

Wang DS, Bennett DA, Mufson EJ, *et al.* (2004). Contribution of changes in ubiquitin and myelin basic protein to age-related cognitive decline. *Neurosci. Res.* **48**:93–100.

Watson GS, Craft S (2003). The role of insulin resistance in the pathogenesis of Alzheimer's disease: implications for treatment. [Review] [163 refs] *CNS Drugs* **17**:27–45.

Chapter 4

Neuropathology of healthy brain aging

Introduction

This chapter describes anatomic changes in the brains of persons who are cognitively normal at the time of death and do not have a recognized neurologic illness.

Certain pathologic conditions such as Alzheimer's disease (AD), senile plaques (SPs), and neurofibrillary tangles (NFTs), and the occurrence of 'incidental' brainstem Lewy bodies, are highly age-associated but are not believed to be *caused by* aging *per se*. The implications of such lesions as possible herald lesions for later development of full-blown disease is discussed in this chapter. Additional discussion may be found in Chapters 5 (on Alzheimer's disease) and 7 (on Parkinson's and related Lewy body disorders).

Pathologists have long appreciated that many systemic disorders are tightly linked to the aging process. Among these are aortic and major vascular systems atherosclerosis (*Box 4.1*, **4.1**) (Roher *et al.*, 2005) and *in situ* carcinoma of

---

Box 4.1 Cerebral atherosclerosis, Alzheimer's disease, and aging

Age is a major risk factor for both cerebral circle of Willis atherosclerosis and Alzheimer senile plaques (SP) (see Chapter 5). The graphs are adapted from a monograph chapter written in 1970 by neuropathologist JAN Corsellis and show the age-related incidences of both types of lesions in an autopsied series of 667 patients from a mental hospital in England. The lesions were graded as less severe (grade 1) and more severe (grades 2 and 3). The incidence of both lesions (y-axis) as percent of cases affected, and severity grades of each, are strikingly related to age at death (x-axis). More modern series based on alpha-beta immunohistochemistry and optimized silver methods for SP would show higher prevalences at the uppermost age ranges. In the authors' experience, more than 90% of persons who die at 90 years or older have some neocortical SP and neurofibrillary tangles in their brains at autopsy. (Adapted from Corsellis, 1970.)

Incidence of atherosclerosis of large cerebral vessels in a series of 667 patients dying in a mental hospital. Light shading shows a slight degree of change (grade 1); dark shading shows changes estimated as moderate to severe (grades 2 or 3).

Incidence of senile plaque formation in the same series as in the previous figure. Light shading shows cases with only a few plaques; dark shading shows those with moderate to severe degrees of plaque formation.

4.1 (**A**) A cross-section of a major cerebral artery shows approximately 30% occlusion of the lumen by a fibrous atherosclerotic plaque (×1 objective). (**B**) Another circle of Willis major arterial tributary shows almost complete occlusion by a fibrofatty atherosclerotic plaque. The latter lesions with 'critical stenosis' (>75% lumenal narrowing) impair blood flow and cause ischemic strokes if sufficient collateral blood supply is not available to meet tissue needs (×1 objective).

Table 4.1 Features of the aging brain

Anatomic lesions	Pathologic lesions
White matter granular degeneration	NFTs in AON, ERC-II, LC, and NBM
Neuronal lipofuscin	Isolated preamyloid and diffuse SP
Corpora amylacea accumulation	CAA
CP calcification	Arterial lipohyalinosis
GFAP mRNA up-regulation	Lacunar infarction
Gracile nucleus neuroaxonal dystrophy	Atherosclerosis of the circle of Willis major arteries
Widened Virchow–Robins spaces reflecting aging-related vascular tortuosity; focal arterial iron/calcium deposition	Hippocampal CA1 GVD (<9% of pyramidal neurons affected)
Localized vertex meningeal fibrosis	Cortical atrophy
Frontal horn rounding (slight)	Ventricular enlargement
Periventricular myelin pallor (MRI and CT 'caps' and 'high signal areas')	Selective neuronal loss (LC, DR, NBM, CA fields of hippocampus, cortex)

the prostate gland in men. When serial sectioning is applied to the prostate glands of autopsied 85-years-olds, Franks (1954) reported that minute latent carcinomatous foci were found in prostate glands of all autopsied men aged 90 years or over. This concept of diseases that are *associated with* but are not caused by aging is important. Brains from persons dying after 90 years of age in the authors' experience, even though normal cognition has been established before death, nevertheless have subthreshold AD lesions that may or may not meet established diagnostic criteria for AD. Nevertheless, the *pattern* of such lesions is often so typical of AD lesion location and distribution as to suggest the presence of a preclinical form of the disease (Arriagada *et al.*, 1992).

Table 4.1 lists the many anatomic and pathologic features that together form the tapestry of the aging healthy brain. While most authorities regard lesions in the left column as benign and without functional consequences, the same is not true for pathologic lesions tabulated in the right column.

Anatomic 'benign' lesions

White matter granular degeneration

In virtually all persons who die after age 50 years, the white matter (WM) exhibits widespread 'granular degeneration' (**4.2**) when stained with an antibody to ubiquitin (Wang *et al.*, 2004). Nearby corpora amylacea (see below) are also ubiquinated. The granules are intimately associated with myelin bundles. The common interpretation among neuropathologists is that this is a universal accompaniment of aging in the human brain. So far, no specific pathologic or functional significance has been attached to the morphologic phenomenon.

Neuronal lipofuscin

Intracellular accumulation of this proteolipid material in secondary lysosomes is a recognized valid correlate of chronological age in both vertebrates and invertebrates (Brunk & Terman, 2002). In the former, lipofuscin pigment accumulates in myocardial cells, hepatocytes, and central neurons (**4.3**). Lipofuscin levels in the superior temporal gyrus do not differ between nondemented controls and AD patients (Mountjoy *et al.*, 2005).

4.2 Ubiquitin antibody localizes to white matter myelin as punctate brown dots, a lesion that is referred to as 'granular degeneration of myelin'. The lesion is almost universal after 50 years of age in persons with no clinically evident neurologic dysfunction. (×40 objective.)

4.3 Nucleus basalis of Meynert cholinergic magnocellular neurons, similar to many others in the human brain, accumulate lipofuscin lipopigment (arrows) as a direct consequence of chronologic aging. The brown pigment represents degraded proteolipids in secondary lysosomes that cannot be entirely digested by acid hydrolases. Lipofuscin pigment appears lighter and finer in texture than neuromelanin, which has a different biochemical composition. (H&E, ×20 objective.)

4.4. Corpora amylacea are round structures formed mostly of glucose polymers. They cluster in white matter around blood vessels, near ependymal surfaces, and at the subpial glia limitans, where formation by astrocytes can be visualized. (H&E, ×20 objective.)

4.5 Choroid plexus blood vessels and connective tissue matrix are prone to develop dystrophic calcification as a function of aging. Such lesions are often visualized as dense areas on MRI and CT brain scans. (H&E, ×1 objective.)

Corpora amylacea (CA)

These bodies of polymerized glucose form in astrocytes and are deposited around ventricular surfaces (**4.4**) (Mrak *et al.*, 1997). CA also occur in the WM fiber tracts and in the subpial membrane. Formerly regarded as completely benign, abnormal CA build-up is now recognized to occur in certain pathologic situations including the temporal lobes of person undergoing resection for intractable temporal lobe epilepsy (Chung & Horoupian, 1996). It has been proposed that CA act as protective traps or sinks for damaged molecules since the core (~4% protein) contains a variety of partly degraded proteins (Cavanagh, 1999). Ubiquitin is a strong biomarker for CA, for example.

Calcification of the choroid plexus (CP)

CP function declines as a function of aging (Rubenstein, 1998); however, the anatomic and biochemical bases for this are not well understood. Neuroradiologists and morphologists are well aware that the CP develops progressive calcification during normal healthy aging (**4.5**). Coincident with interstitial calcification, CP arteries exhibit collagen fibrous replacement, often referred to as 'hyalinization', of their walls.

Ferruginization of cerebral arteries

Cerebral arteries in the basal ganglia, thalamus, and cerebellar WM are prone to develop mural deposits of calcium and iron with aging (**4.6**). Usually this is a focal and incidental finding of no established clinical significance. It is unclear why these particular blood vessels develop dystrophic calcification and iron deposition. Small arteries and arterioles in the end plate region of the hippocampus also occasionally become calcified in a similar fashion.

Up-regulation of the glial acid fibrillary protein (GFAP) messenger RNA and protein

A number of studies have documented that GFAP mRNA and the GFAP intermediate filament protein of astrocytes are up-regulated during normal aging in the mouse and human brain (Nichols *et al.*, 1993). The precise biochemical basis for this change is not known. It is possible that GFAP increases as part of a general 'gliosis' that accompanies multifocal neuronal loss but this theory has not yet been substantiated. Gliosis is further discussed in Chapter 5 (**5.21**; Schechter *et al.*, 1981).

4.6 Arteries in the thalamus, cerebellum, and basal ganglia such as this one in the nucleus accumbens accumulate aging-associated dystrophic mural deposits of calcium and iron salts that may be visualized with ordinary H&E or Perl's iron stain. (×20 objective.)

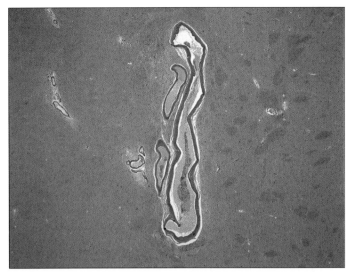

4.7 A deep white collection of blood vessel profiles is consistent with a three dimensional tortuous course, where vascular loops have been cross-sectioned several times within a 6 μm histologic section (see Nonaka *et al.*, 2003). (H&E, ×1 objective.)

Widening of Virchow–Robins perivascular spaces

Nonaka *et al.* (1993) have shown a dramatic increase in WM vascular tortuosity in the aging brain. In fact, micro-angiographic studies combined with scanning electron microscopy have shown that certain blood vessels develop twisted pretzel-like 'knots.' The consequence is a widening of the surrounding perivascular spaces to accommodate the widened vascular loops. This change can be detected in ordinary H&E sections (**4.7**).

The posterior subputamenal region brain is often the site of dramatically widened Virchow–Robins spaces seen by magnetic resonance imaging (MRI) and on gross examination. Experienced neuroradiologists recognize these lesions as a normal anatomic variant, but less experienced diagnosticians may occasionally mistake large ones for lacunar infarcts or small hemorrhagic foci.

Meningeal fibrosis

The leptomeninges at the vertex of the cerebral hemispheres develop aging-related circumscribed collagen fibrosis that conforms to the area bounded when the touching thumbs and middle fingers of both hands are placed over the vertex (**4.8**). This can be a useful 'rule of thumb' guideline since meningeal fibrosis may be mistaken at autopsy for purulent exudate indicative of an acute bacterial meningitis.

4.8 The dorsum of brains of individuals beyond age 40 years progressively develop localized fibrous opacification of the meninges over the vertex of the cerebrum as a function of aging. This normal finding should not be confused with the accumulation of yellow-green purulent material in cases of acute bacterial meningitis.

Frontal horn ventricular rounding

Experience observing more than 1,020 histologically studied brains from nondemented and demented individuals in the Alzheimer's Disease Research Center (ADRC) registry provide convincing evidence that pathologic ventricular enlargement in persons with mild AD is often labeled as 'ventricular enlargement appropriate for age' by radiologists. The intent appears to be to not unduly alarm patients but this may be misleading and unfair as evidence continues to build that medial temporal and frontal atrophy occur early in the course of AD, including the preclinical phase (Fotenos *et al.*, 2005). Good intentions do not necessarily make good science! A better approach would be to develop (or apply existing) objective criteria for scoring brain atrophy and ventricular dilatation and to apply them routinely to structural MRI scans on nondemented elderly persons. The author developed one such method with neuroradiologist Mokhtar Gado, MD (see *Box 5.3*, p. 80) (McKeel & Gado, 1994), and a parallel method was developed for antemortem MRI structural studies with cognitive neuropsychologist Randy Buckner, PhD, at Washington University (*Box 4.2*).

Periventricular myelin pallor (scan 'caps' and 'high signal areas')

Brain scans (computed tomography [CT], MRI) from elderly nondemented patients frequently reveal WM lesions (WMLs) that are both periventricular and deep. An exact histopathologic correlate of these often dramatic MRI appearances has not emerged. Periventricular 'caps' on MRI correspond to areas that by H&E screening stain and LFB-PAS myelin stain conform to WM areas of 'pallor' where myelinated fibers are spread apart, may be pale, and are frequently associated with thickened blood vessels with hyalinized acellular walls (Morris *et al.*, 1990). Inflammatory cells and macrophages are usually inconspicuous in such areas. Many investigators believe the primary lesion in such areas of pallor is focal cerebral edema. Subependymal blood vessels, for example in the caudate nucleus, undergo similar hyaline mural thickening surrounded by widened perivascular spaces (**4.9**).

Deeper mild WMLs may show edema or a lesion that Brun and Englund called 'incomplete infarction' (1986). Besides edema and pallor, WM contains some macrophages and a diminished number of oligodendrocytes, which the

---

Box 4.2 MRI brain atrophy and aging

Structural T1 weighted brain magnetic resonance image (MRI) scans provide excellent anatomic correlation during life with postmortem atrophy scores (compare with *Box 5.3*, p. 80). Gray and white matter and the cerebral ventricular system size may be assessed. Row 1 includes MRI images from a normal college-aged person. The angles of the frontal horns are razor sharp (left column), the body of the ventricle is small (middle column), and the ventricular trigone (right column) is also very small. The middle and lower rows display progressive degrees of cerebral atrophy and ventricular dilatation seen in Alzheimer patients. The number to the left is the atrophy/ventricular size score to compare with the anatomic visual standards (*Box 5.3*, p. 80). Grades 2 and 3 show progressive gyral gray matter thinning, sulcal widening, hippocampal atrophy, and white matter loss in addition to the ventricular size alterations.

Frontal horns   Body and   Trigone
                     temporal horns

Scandinavian authors believe represent subinfarctive ischemic lesions. Acceptance of the incomplete infarction theory of deep WMLs is not universal because several careful studies in which lesion-bearing MRI regions were examined histologically have shown only edema rather than tissue ischemic necrosis (Scheltens *et al.*, 1995). In addition, clinical stroke history has been reported to correlate poorly with WMLs on MRI or CT scans.

From this pathologist's experience, the overwhelming majority of WMLs seen on MRI appear to represent WM edema primarily when the brain is viewed at autopsy. Grossly, no pathology is seen in the usual case regardless of the 'severity' (number, spatial extent) of the WMLs. The exception at the microscopic level is that periventricular blood vessels in the regions of MRI WM 'caps' have thickened, acellular, fibrotic ('hyaline change') walls (**4.10**). This vascular change is almost universal after about age 50 years. The age when this fibrohyalinosis of periventricular vasculature begins has not yet been precisely defined.

Pathologic lesions

Aging related neurofibrillary tangles (NFTs) in selected brain regions

Evidence exists that NFTs occur in certain brain regions: entorhinal cortex layer II (ERC-II) (Price *et al.*, 1991), nucleus basalis of Meynert (NBM) (Beach *et al.*, 1998), locus ceruleus (LC) (DW McKeel, Jr, unpublished data), and anterior olfactory nucleus (AON) (Price *et al.*, 1991), as a function of normal aging in the absence of Alzheimer type plaques (**4.11**). The work group that formulated the National Institute on Aging (NIA)-Reagan Institute criteria for diagnosing AD (1997) stated that even a single NFT should be regarded as pathologic. The real issue is whether or not NFTs occur as isolated lesions as an integral part of the aging process, or, are NFTs in the above regions a harbinger of AD that appears in a discordant temporal sequence before the appearance of SPs in the neocortex?

Experience at the authors' ADRC confirms that a few

4.9 Subependymal (lumen at the left) blood vessel walls, difficult to identify as either arteries or veins, in aging brains are routinely acellular with thickened fibrous walls. (H&E, ×10 objective.)

4.10 A deep centrum semiovale white matter blood vessel shows remarkable thickening and dense, nearly acellular walls that consist of collagen bundles. The process is similar to that shown in **4.9**, but is more extreme. (H&E, ×10 objective.)

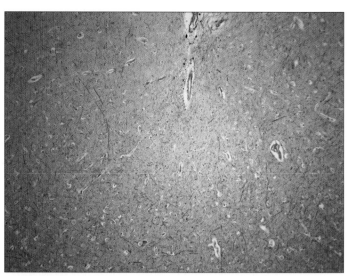

4.11 Isolated argyrophilic neurofibrillary tangles are a common autopsy finding in the nucleus basalis of Meynert after age 50 years, even in nondemented persons. The nearby neuronal population appears normal. (Modified Bielschowsky silver method, ×20 objective.)

4.12 A silver stain fails to show any senile plaques or neurofibrillary tangles in the superior temporal cerebral neocortex of this 86-year-old nondemented man. (Modified Bielschowsky silver method, ×10 objective.)

tangles are often seen in ERC-II, NBM, AON, LC, and the substantia nigra (SN) of nondemented controls that are rated CDR 0 at death. Neuropil threads (NT) co-occur in small numbers with NFTs in ERC-II, LC, and SN (Braak *et al.*, 1986).

Isolated preamyloid and diffuse senile plaques

The most controversial issue in diagnosing Alzheimer's disease using pathologic criteria is the clinical importance of non-neuritic senile plaques (NNSPs) in the brains of nondemented elderly individuals. Extensive data on nondemented elderly brains has been obtained at the authors' center (Price & Morris, 1999 [39 brains]; Morris *et al.*, 1996 [21 brains]; Price *et al.*, 2001 [39 brains]; DW McKeel, Jr and NS Havlioglu 'decades study' [104 institutional controls, unpublished data]) and in collaboration with six other ADRCs (Morris *et al.*, 2004). These studies collectively indicate there are three basic classes of AD type neuropathology that characterize nondemented aging as described below.

About 60% of brains from persons who are 70 years or more at death have no demonstrable argyrophilic (silver positive) or a-beta immunoreactive (Aβ-IR) plaque-like deposits in either the neocortex (**4.12**) or hippocampus. The

stellate neurons that comprise the ERC-II and the most medial segment of hippocampal CA1 (the 'initial segment') almost always contain a few neurofibrillary pretangles and intraneuronal tangles that are staged as Braak I–II (Braak and Braak, 1991). In the authors' experience NFTs in ERC-II and CA1 are first seen during the sixth decade (50–60 years) (NS Havlioglu and DW McKeel, Jr, unpublished data). Persons dying at younger ages may have no demonstrable NFTs in the same brain regions (Braak stage 0).

A few SPs may be detected using a-beta antibodies and the Hedreen–Bielschowsky silver method in many brains with zero or only a few isolated NFTs (**4.13**). These are the authors' ADRC's most sensitive lesion detection methods. Thus, NFTs rarely occur in total isolation in the vulnerable regions discussed in this chapter. SP burden, however, may be very low and individual SPs or small SP clusters may be spread far apart in the voluminous, highly folded cerebral cortex. Preamyloid SPs (Tagliavini *et al.*, 1988) by definition are labeled with a-beta antibodies but fail to stain with silver, thioflavine S, or Congo red. As a result, unless a-beta immunohistochemistry is used, preamyloid plaques that precede, or coincide with, formation of both diffuse and neuritic SPs will fail to be detected.

A minority (25–40%, Morris *et al.*, 2004) of brains from

4.13 The superior temporal cortex of a 87-year-old nondemented man displays patchy diffuse senile plaques (SP) in both modified Bielschowsky silver (**A**) and amyloid beta (a-beta) immunohistochemical stains (brown peroxidase substrate) (**B**). In contrast to diffuse SP, preamyloid plaques, had they been present, would stain only with a-beta antibody but not with silver methods. (×10 objective for both panels.)

nondemented elderly persons 70–100+ years of age at death have both SPs and NFTs in the distribution pattern that characterizes brains from very mildly cognitively impaired (i.e. CDR 0.5) AD patients and persons with mild cognitive impairment (MCI) in the memory domain (**4.14**) (Petersen, 2004). The authors regard these people as having preclinical AD since 70% will progress to mild (CDR 1) AD within 2 years (Goldman *et al.*, 2001). The detailed presentation of preclinical pathologic AD is contained in Chapter 5 on the neuropathology of clinically overt AD.

One may wonder why it appears so difficult for pathologists to agree on a universal definition of AD in all its stages. Pathologists commonly examine one histologic section with a dimension of approximately 0.8 inches × 0.8 inches × 6 μm thick for each cerebral lobe. One to four such sections thus routinely constitutes the 'neocortical' sample. Accordingly, small numbers of cortical plaques or isolated tangles (or any other dispersed lesion) could be easily missed using such a sampling scheme. It is therefore the authors' opinion that 'isolated' tangles and sparse SP may constitute the earliest demonstrable lesion profile of the earliest anatomic expression of AD. A high density unbiased sampling study would be necessary to determine more definitively whether SPs or NFTs appear first.

4.14 Prefrontal cortex of an 82-year-old very mildly demented (CDR 0.5) woman contains widespread dense beta-amyloid deposits but only rare neurofibrillary tau-positive tangles or tau-positive neuropil threads. (Dual immunohistochemistry with antibodies to beta amyloid [red substrate] and hyperphosphorylated tau [blue-black substrate], ×10 objective.)

4.15 Leptomeningeal large and smaller arteries of this 90-year-old woman stain intensely with beta-amyloid antibody and a red substrate. (Dual immuno-histochemistry with antibodies to beta amyloid [red substrate] and hyperphosphorylated tau [blue-black substrate], ×10 objective.)

4.16 A deep white matter artery shows mural thickening with prominent outer medial and adventitial fibrosis, the so-called lipohyaline change. Such vessels often display perivascular hemosiderin macrophages, indicating bleeding has occurred. A few chronic inflammatory cells are also commonly present around such arteries. (H&E, ×20 objective.)

Isolated cerebral amyloid angiopathy (CAA)

Focal deposits of a-beta peptide in leptomeningeal arteries are relatively common in brains of nondemented elderly persons (**4.15**). The occurrence rate is 10–30% in various reported series (Revesz *et al.*, 2003). The reported prevalence of CAA is partly influenced by the method used to detect vascular amyloid. Precise comparative performance data of Congo red, thioflavine S, Gallyas silver, and a-beta immunohistochemistry to detect CAA are not available. In the authors' experience, Congo red is least sensitive, while the other three methods have roughly comparable sensitivity to detect cerebral beta amyloid deposits. The fact that elderly persons with isolated CAA developed lobar cerebral hemorrhages (Izumihara *et al.*, 2005) is evidence that CAA, in the absence of AD, is a potentially serious condition rather than being a benign lesion. CAA should also be regarded as aging-associated rather than being a direct effect of aging. This interpretation is supported by the fact that a large majority of elderly persons do not have demonstrable CAA in routine autopsy brain sections.

Arterial lipohyalinosis

Cerebral arteries undergo a series of histopathologic changes as part of normal aging. These changes must be distinguished from the effects of vascular risk factors, most importantly hypertension and diabetes mellitus. The vascular wall of certain blood vessels may lose smooth muscle cells and undergo replacement fibrosis (**4.16**) (Thal *et al.*, 2003). Arterial lipohyalinosis is a more specific vascular lesion that is exacerbated by hypertension and aging. Affected arteries develop foamy macrophages as well as fibrosis.

Lacunar infarction

No one doubts that small lacunar infarcts (<1.5 cm as originally described by CM Fisher [1965]) are pathologic lesions. However, they are so common in certain regions such as the thalamus, caudate, and putamen that some regard them as 'aging'-related lesions. The detailed gross and microscopic pathology of lacunar infarcts is covered in Chapter 6 on lesions that are associated with vascular dementia.

4.17 A coronal section through the brain of a 90-year-old female (CDR 0.5 at death, apolipoprotein E genotype ε24) had 19 macroscopically identifiable infarcts throughout her cerebrum. The arrows point to small infarcts in both caudate nuclei and a part of the inferior temporal cortex. (Formalin fixed autopsy specimen.)

4.18 A coronal slide 1 cm behind **4.17** reveals large infarcts that destroyed the right hypothalamus. The opposite putamen has a large slit-like infarct. The cortex also has a small infarct (arrows). (Formalin fixed autopsy specimen.)

A case example illustrates why interpretation of small vascular lesions in the aging brain is so difficult. A 90-year-old woman had very mild CDR 0.5 dementia during life but had 19 discrete infarcts in her brain at autopsy (**4.17**). Her apolipoprotien E (apoE) genotype was 24. Sparse neocortical diffuse SPs were detected (see **4.13**). One such lesion destroyed the hypothalamus and one mammillary body (**4.18**), and probably contributed to her death. Microscopic examination revealed both focal subacute lesions with gitter macrophages and perilesional reactive astrocytosis (**4.19**), together with small remote cavitary lesions.

4.19 A small, sharply defined white matter subacute infarct is characterized by tissue destruction with loss of both myelin and axons. The demarcating cavity is filled with foamy macrophages ('gitter' cells). Had this lesion progressed, a cavitary 'lacune' would have ensued. (H&E, ×10 objective.)

4.20 The arterial circle of Willis has been dissected away from the base of the brain at autopsy. The anterior circulation is at left and the posterior vertebrobasilar circulation is at right. Note the preferential involvement of anterior arteries by yellow nonoccluding atherosclerotic plaques. The autopsy specimen is from the same patient's brain portrayed in **4.18** and **4.19**.

4.21 This high magnification image shows hippocampal CA1 neurons with two distinct age-associated lesions. Granulovacuolar degeneration (yellow arrow) presents as cytoplasmic clear zones containing a denser granule. Such regions of the cell sequester tubulin and caspase-3 as well as other cytoskeletal elements (autophagocytosis). The three black arrows point to individual Hirano bodies, actin paracrystalline lattices that form within, and are enveloped by, neuronal plasma membranes. Both lesions increase in number and spatial distribution in Alzheimer's disease compared to normal aging (see Woodard, 1962; Fisher, 1965; Selznick *et al.*, 1999). (H&E, x40 objective.)

Atherosclerosis of the arterial circle of Willis

Atherosclerosis is a pathologic aging-associated process whereby foamy lipid-rich macrophages and smooth muscle cells build up in the walls of large cerebral arteries. The arterial circle of Willis at the base of the brain and its arterial tributaries develop segmental, regional, and diffuse disease (**4.20**). Such atherosclerotic plaques, when the lumen is compromised greater than about 75%, may lead to occlusive reductions of blood flow (see **4.1**). The result is either transient infarction with minimal or no lasting clinical sequelae (transient ischemic attacks, TIAs), or completed ischemic infarcts (strokes) with permanent destruction of brain tissue. Atherosclerosis and infarction are discussed in more depth in Chapter 6 on the pathology of cerebro-vascular dementia.

Hippocampal CA1 granulovacuolar degeneration (GVD)

Pyramidal neuronal cells of the hippocampal CA1 field develop a cytoplasmic lesion termed GVD that consists of a clear vacuole, in the center of which is a dense granule (**4.21**). The dense granules are labeled with antibodies to tubulin, tau, and activated caspase-3 (Selznick *et al.*, 1999). Two studies (Woodard, 1962; Tomlinson and Kitchener, 1972) have shown that up to 9% of CA1 neurons may be affected in nondemented individuals. In contrast, they as well as Ball (1978) have shown that GVD prevalences higher than 9% are strongly correlated with NFTs and related AD pathologic lesions.

4.22 Superior temporal neocortex from a 91-year-old apolipoprotein E ε33 genotype woman shows nearly normal appearing neuronal and glial histology, even though she was moderately demented at the time of death. (H&E, ×10 objective.)

Cortical atrophy

Dekaban showed in 1978, based on autopsy brain weights of over 2,400 men and 2,300 women, that the human brains loses mass at the rate of about 0.2% per decade beginning at age 50–55 years. Modern MRI volumetric studies have confirmed that cortical gray matter loss occurs at about this same rate in nondemented persons as a function of age. Atrophy rates that are higher may herald the presence of incipient dementia (Fotenos *et al.*, 2005), as discussed further in Chapter 5 on the neuropathology of preclinical and overt AD.

Ventricular enlargement

Data from Kaye's group (Mueller *et al.*, 1998) and from the authors' center indicate that cognitively defined persons who are CDR 0 have near normal sized cerebral ventricular systems through their 90s. Coronal sections reveal slight rounding of the frontal horn lateral angles, mild enlargement of the temporal horns with slight hippocampal atrophy, and near normal sized ventricular bodies and trigonal areas. Such brains are represented in row 1 of *Box 4.2*. When greater degrees of sulcal widening and ventricular enlargement are encountered as shown in rows 2 and 3 of *Box 4.2*, an incipient or established dementing disorder should be suspected as the underlying cause.

Selective neuronal loss

Studies by Brody (1955) and others indicated that perhaps 50% of cortical neurons were lost as part of normal brain aging. Beginning in the 1970s with quantitative image analysis studies and continuing with the application of unbiased stereologic quantification of human neuronal populations, it has become clear that age-associated neuronal loss in the human brain is highly selective and certainly is of lesser overall magnitude than the Brody studies had indicated (**4.22**). For example, quantitative morphometric analysis indicates that LC pigmented noradrenergic neurons are lost during aging (Lohr & Jeste, 1988), whereas superior temporal sulcus (Gómez-Isla *et al.*, 1997) and ERC-II (Gómez-Isla *et al.*, 1996) and hippocampal CA1 neurons are well maintained in cognitively intact persons up to their 90s (Price *et al.*, 2001).

As will be seen in the following chapter on AD, the borderline between normal healthy brain aging and early AD dementing disease is still being defined clinically, psychometrically, by neuroimaging modalities, and by neuropathology. This challenging task is hindered by a lack of precise criteria for diagnosing the earliest manifestations of AD.

References

Arriagada PV, Marzloff K, Hyman BT (1992). Distribution of Alzheimer-type pathologic changes in nondemented elderly individuals matches the pattern in Alzheimer's disease. *Neurology* **42**:1681–1688.

Ball MJ (1978). Topographic distribution of neurofibrillary tangles and granulovacuolar degeneration in hippocampal cortex of aging and demented patients. A quantitative study. *Acta Neuropathol* **42**:73–80.

Beach TG, Sue LI, Scott S, et al. (1998). Neurofibrillary tangles are constant in aging human nucleus basalis. *Alzheimer's Rep.* **6**:375–380.

Braak H, Braak E (1991). The neuropathologic stageing of Alzheimer-related changes. *Acta Neuropathol.* (Berlin) **82**:239–259.

Braak H, Braak E, Grundke-Iqbal I, et al. (1986). Occurrence of neuropil threads in the senile human brain and in Alzheimer's disease: a third location of paired helical filaments outside of neurofibrillary tangles and neuritic plaques. *Neurosci. Lett.* **65**:351–355.

Brody H (1955). Organization of the cerebral cortex. III. A study of aging in the human cerebral cortex. *J. Comp. Neurol.* **102**:511–516.

Brun A, Englund E (1986). A white matter disorder in dementia of the Alzheimer type: a pathoanatomical study. *Ann. Neurol.* **19**:253–262.

Brunk UT, Terman A (2002). Lipofuscin: mechanisms of age-related accumulation and influence on cell function. (Review) (75 refs). *Free Radical Biology & Medicine* **33**:611–619.

Cavanagh JB (1999). Corpora amylacea and the family of polyglucosan diseases. (Review) (235 refs). *Brain Res. Rev.* **29**:265–295.

Chung MH. Horoupian DS (1996). Corpora amylacea: a marker for mesial temporal sclerosis. *J. Neuropathol. Exp. Neurol.* **55**:403–408.

Dekaban AS (1978). Changes in brain weights during the span of human life: relation of brain weights to body heights and body weights. *Ann. Neurol.* **4**:345–356.

Fisher CM (1965). Lacune: small deep cerebral infarcts. *Neurology* **15**:774–784.

Fotenos AF, Snyder AZ, Girton LE, et al. (2005). Normative estimates of cross-sectional and longitudinal brain volume decline in aging and AD. *Neurology* **64**:1032–1039.

Franks LM (1954). Latent carcinoma of the prostate. *J. Pathol. Bacteriol.* **68**:603–616.

Goldman WP, Storandt M, Miller JP, et al. (2001). Mild cognitive impairment represents early-stage Alzheimer's disease. *Arch. Neurol.* **58**:397–405.

Gómez-Isla T, Hollister R, West H, et al. (1997). Neuronal loss correlates with but exceeds neurofibrillary tangles in Alzheimer's disease. *Ann. Neurol.* **41**:17–24.

Gómez-Isla T, Price JL, McKeel DW Jr, et al. (1996). Profound loss of layer II entorhinal cortex neurons in very mild Alzheimer's disease. *J. Neurosci.* **16**:4491–4500.

Izumihara A, Suzuki M, Ishihara T (2005). Recurrence and extension of lobar hemorrhage related to cerebral amyloid angiopathy: multivariate analysis of clinical risk factors. *Surg. Neurol.* **64**:160–164.

Lohr JB, Jeste DV (1988). Locus ceruleus morphometry in aging and schizophrenia. (Review) (48 refs). *Acta Psych. Scand.* **77**:689–697.

McKeel DW Jr, Gado M (1994). A visual standards based system for scoring Alzheimer and aging-related human brain atrophy at autopsy (abstr. P34-11). *Brain Pathol.* **4**:544.

Morris JC, Gado M, Torack RM, et al. (1990). Binswanger's disease or artifact: a clinical, neuroimaging, and pathological study of periventricular white matter changes in Alzheimer's disease. *Adv. Neurol.* **51**:47–52.

Morris JC, Hurst E, McKeel DW Jr, et al. (2000). Healthy brain aging in nonagenarians and centenarians. *World Congress of Neurology* July.

Morris JC, McKeel DW Jr, Buckles VD, et al. (2004). Neuropathological markers of preclinical Alzheimer's disease in nondemented aging. *J. Neurosci. Abstr.* **902**:16; online (URL: http://sfn.scholarone.com/itin2004/index.html).

Morris JC, Storandt M, McKeel DW Jr, et al. (1996). Cerebral amyloid deposition and diffuse plaques in 'normal' aging: evidence for presymptomatic and very mild Alzheimer's disease. *Neurology* **46**:707–719.

Mountjoy CQ, Dowson JH, Harrington C, et al. (2005). Characteristics of neuronal lipofuscin in the superior temporal gyrus in Alzheimer's disease do not differ from nondiseased controls: a comparison with disease-related changes in the superior frontal gyrus. *Acta Neuropathol.* **109**:490–496.

Mrak RE, Griffin ST, Graham DI 91997). Aging-associated changes in human brain. (Review) (60 refs). *J. Neuropathol. Exp. Neurol.* **56**:1269–1275.

Mueller EA, Moore MM, Kerr DC, *et al.* (1998). Brain volume preserved in healthy elderly through the eleventh decade. *Neurology* **51**:1555–1562.

NIA-Reagan Institute Working Group on Diagnostic Criteria for Neuropathological Assessment of Alzheimer's disease (1997). Working Group consensus recommendations for the postmortem diagnosis of Alzheimer's disease. *Neurobiol. Aging* **18**(Suppl 4):S1–S2.

Nichols NR, Day JR, Laping NJ, *et al.* (1993). GFAP mRNA increases with age in rat and human brain. *Neurobiol Aging* **14**:421–429.

Nonaka H, Akima M, Hatori T, *et al.* (2003). The microvasculature of the cerebral white matter: arteries of the subcortical white matter. *J. Neuropathol. Exp. Neurol.* **62**:154–161.

Petersen RC (2004). Mild cognitive impairment as a diagnostic entity. (Review) (50 refs). *J. Int. Med.* **256**:183–194.

Price JL, Davis PB, Morris JC, *et al.* (1991). The distribution of tangles, plaques and related immunohistochemical markers in healthy aging and Alzheimer's disease. *Neurobiol. Aging* **12**:295–312.

Price JL, Ko AI, Wade MJ, *et al.* (2001). Neuron number in entorhinal cortex and CA1 in preclinical Alzheimer's disease. *Arch. Neurol.* **58**:1395–1402.

Price JL, Morris JC (1999). Tangles and plaques in nondemented aging and 'preclinical' Alzheimer's disease. *Ann. Neurol.* **51**:47–52.

Revesz T, Ghiso J, Lashley T, *et al.* (2003). Cerebral amyloid angiopathies: a pathologic, biochemical, and genetic view. (Review) (80 refs). *J. Neuropathol. Exp. Neurol.* **62**:885–898.

Roher AE, Esh C, Rahman A, *et al.* (2005). Atherosclerosis of cerebral arteries in Alzheimer disease. *Stroke* **35**(Suppl 1):2623–2627.

Rubenstein E (1998). Relationship of senescence of cerebrospinal fluid circulatory system to dementias of the aged. (Review) (32 refs). *Lancet* **351**:283–285.

Scheltens P, Barkhof F, Leys D, *et al.* (1995). Histopathologic correlates of white matter changes on MRI in Alzheimer's disease and normal aging. *Neurology* **45**:883–888.

Selznick LA, Holtzman DM, Han BH, *et al.* (1999). *In situ* immunodetection of neuronal caspase-3 activation in Alzheimer disease. *J. Neuropathol. Exp. Neurol.* **58**:1020–1026.

Tagliavini F, Giaccone G, Frangione B, *et al.* (1988). Preamyloid deposits in the cerebral cortex of patients with Alzheimer's disease and nondemented individuals. *Neurosci. Lett.* **93**:191–196.

Thal DR, Ghebremedhin E, Orantes M, *et al.* (2003). Vascular pathology in Alzheimer disease: correlation of cerebral amyloid angiopathy and arteriosclerosis/lipo-hyalinosis with cognitive decline. *J. Neuropathol. Exp. Neurol.* **62**:1287–1301.

Tomlinson BE, Kitchener D (1972). Granulovacuolar degeneration of hippocampal pyramidal cells. *J. Pathol.* **106**:165–185.

Wang DS, Bennett DA, Mufson EJ, *et al.* (2004). Contribution of changes in ubiquitin and myelin basic protein to age-related cognitive decline. *Neurosci. Res.* **48**:93–100.

Woodard JS (1962). Clinicopathologic significance of granulovacuolar degeneration in Alzheimer's disease. *J. Neuropathol. Exp. Neurol.* **21**:85–91.

Chapter 5

Neuropathology of preclinical and clinical Alzheimer's disease

Introduction

Alzheimer's disease (AD) represents a tremendous public health burden as it accounts for 50–70% of cases of dementia and is by far the most common form of dementia. 20 million individuals worldwide are afflicted with AD, 4 million in the US. Incident cases of AD are expected to nearly triple in the US over the next 50 years (Hebert *et al.*, 2001). As the prevalence of AD doubles every 5 years after the age of 65 years, reaching nearly 50% in those aged over 85 years (Ebly *et al.*, 1994), the significance of AD worldwide will only increase as life expectancy improves and the population ages.

Clinical features

Table 5.1 presents the common symptoms of early AD. Short-term memory impairment is the hallmark of early AD. Common early manifestations of memory decline include forgetfulness of recent conversations, repetition of questions, and missing appointments. Early memory impairment is often accompanied by executive dysfunction leading to problems in planning and organizing. These cognitive deficits are responsible for progressive impairment in activities of daily living such as driving, shopping, managing finances, and cooking. With disease progression, impairment in other cognitive domains such as language,

Table 5.1 Common symptoms of early Alzheimer's disease

Memory loss
- Forgetful of pertinent details of recent events
- Repeating questions
- Misplacement of items

Executive dysfunction
- Difficulties managing checkbook/household finances
- Decline in cooking skills
- Decline in home repair/maintenance skills
- Trouble operating household appliances (microwave, TV remote control, telephone)

Daily activities
- Impaired performance in hobbies (playing cards, reading)
- Difficulty driving (getting lost, indecisiveness, minor or major accidents)
- Shopping (frequent trips for forgotten items, doubling up on items)

visuospatial function, calculations, and praxis becomes apparent. AD results in progressive disability, dependency, and eventually death. The mean survival after AD symptom onset is 10.3 years but may range from 2 to more than 20 years (Mendez & Cummings, 2003).

Clinical diagnostic criteria

While confirmation of the diagnosis of AD rests on neuropathologic observations after death, increasing knowledge about the clinical and behavioral symptoms of AD have improved the ability to identify AD with high accuracy (90% or higher in autopsy confirmed series from dementia research centers) (Berg *et al.*, 1998). The diagnosis of AD has been standardized with criteria developed by the Work Group of the National Institute of Neurologic and Communicative Disorders and Stroke and the Alzheimer's Disease and Related Disorders Association (NINCDS-ADRDA).

The NINCDS-ADRDA criteria (McKhann *et al.*, 1984) established three levels of confidence for the diagnosis of AD: probable, possible, and definite (*Table 5.2*). Definite AD can only be diagnosed by autopsy. Probable AD is diagnosed 'if there is a typical insidious onset of dementia with progression and if there are no other systemic or brain diseases that could account for the progressive memory and other cognitive deficits'. Possible AD is diagnosed when there are variations in the presentation or course of dementia, such as early or disproportionate language disturbance, or when another potentially dementing disorder (e.g. stroke) is present but is not believed to be responsible for dementia. The development of standard clinical criteria has led to rapid advances in the clinicopathologic study of AD and the implementation of multi-center clinical trials.

Table 5.2 NINCDS–ADRDA criteria for Alzheimer's disease (AD)

Probable AD
- Measurable deficits in two or more areas of cognition
- No disturbance in consciousness
- Progressive worsening
- Onset between 40 and 90 years
- Absence of systemic disease or other brain disease that could account for the deficits
- Diagnostic support:
  – Progressive deterioration
  – Impaired ADLs
  – Family history of similar disorder
  – Normal LP/EEG
  – Atrophy on CT
- Other consistent clinical features include plateaus in the course of progression, associated symptoms of depression, insomnia, incontinence, delusions, illusions, sexual disorders, seizures (in advanced disease), neurologic abnormalities such as increased tone, myoclonus, gait disorders

- Features making diagnosis unlikely include sudden onset, focal neurologic signs, seizures or gait disturbance early in the course

Possible AD
- Dementia syndrome with variations in onset, course, or presentation or the presence of other problems or disorders that may produce dementia but are not considered the cause of dementia

Definite AD
- Clinical criteria met
- Histopathologic evidence present at autopsy

ADL: activities of daily living; CT: computed tomography; EEG: electroencephalogram; LP: lumbar puncture.

(McKhann *et al.*, 1984)

Evaluation of suspected AD

The evaluation of dementia consists of a combination of five components: history taking, physical examination, psychometric testing, neuroimaging, and laboratory testing.

History

The key information needed to diagnose dementia and create a differential diagnosis comes primarily from the clinical information. Clinically diagnosing AD rests on determining whether cognitive decline is present to such a degree as to interfere with function in usual activities. Observations from an attentive family member, relative, or friend describing cognitive changes interfering even mildly with the patient's usual function are essential in making a confident diagnosis.

Physical examination

In mild and even moderate AD, focal neurologic abnormalities are infrequent. The neurologic exam is performed primarily to evaluate for the presence of any signs suggestive of another dementing illness such as focal upper motor neuron signs, extrapyramidal signs, and prominent aphasia and apraxia (*Table 5.3*). Focal neurologic deficits may indicate the presence of significant vascular disease, which commonly coexists with AD, and may play a role in the symptomatic expression of AD (Snowdon *et al.*, 1997). The presence of increased tone and a Parkinsonian gait early

in the course may indicate dementia with Lewy bodies or Parkinson's dementia. Extrapyramidal signs are common in advanced AD but are generally not prominent early in the course. Prominent unilateral extrapyramidal signs may indicate corticobasal degeneration. Prominent myoclonus may indicate Creutzfeldt–Jakob disease, especially if accompanying a rapidly progressive dementing illness, although myoclonus can also be encountered in AD.

Psychometric testing

Mental status tests should be used primarily to confirm the presence of cognitive deficits and not as a method of diagnosis. Mental status tests cannot, certainly at the initial evaluation, indicate whether the individual has declined from previous levels of cognitive abilities nor determine the presence of impairment sufficient to interfere with accustomed activities. Testing is useful in demonstrating a pattern of deficits consistent with an AD pattern (primary deficits in memory and executive function) and to monitor dementia progression over time through serial testing. Over-reliance on cognitive test performance in addition to failure to incorporate an informant's observations about an individual's cognitive function in relation to past abilities results in the under-recognition of mild AD.

Neuroimaging

Structural neuroimaging is recommended in the form of either magnetic resonance imaging (MRI) or noncontrast computed tomography (CT). The basis of this recommendation is evidence that up to 5% of patients with dementia have a clinically significant structural lesion that would not have been predicted based on the history or examination (Chui & Zhang, 1997). These potential lesions include brain neoplasms, subdural hematomas, or normal pressure hydrocephalus. However, fully reversible dementia due to unsuspected causes is rare.

A number of techniques are being explored in an attempt to identify inclusionary neuroimaging findings to support the diagnosis of AD. A major thrust has been in identifying neuroanatomic changes, such as atrophy, that may predict cognitive decline related to AD. The molecular imaging of amyloid deposits has promise as a potential biomarker for AD, and possibly may allow the identification of individuals who are still in the presymptomatic stages of the illness (*Box 5.1*, overleaf).

Table 5.3 Features suggestive of other dementing illness

Parkinsonism: dementia with Lewy bodies, corticobasal degeneration

Language:
- Naming impairment: progressive nonfluent aphasia
- Comprehension impairment: semantic dementia

Apraxia: corticobasal degeneration

Myoclonus: prion disease (Creutzfeldt–Jakob disease)

Box 5.1 Imaging amyloid

The molecular imaging of amyloid deposits has promise as a potential biomarker for AD and possibly may allow the identification of individuals who are still in the presymptomatic stages of the illness (Mintun *et al.*, 2006). Radioligands have been developed that cross the blood–brain barrier and bind specifically to amyloid aggregates in sufficient amounts to be imaged by PET (Revesz *et al.*, 2003; Attems & Jellinger, 2004). These images demonstrate increased uptake of the radioligand as evident by increased signal detected using PET imaging (yellow and red signal) in an individual with AD (**A**) compared to an individual without cognitive decline (**B**). (Adapted from Mintun *et al.*, 2006).

In a proof of concept PET study, a benzothiole amyloid agent, also known as Pittsburgh compound-B (PIB), resulted in significantly higher standardized uptake values in 16 AD patients compared to 6 elderly control subjects in regions known to have extensive amyloid deposition (Izumihara *et al.*, 2005). Preferential retention of PIB in frontal and temporoparietal cortex discriminated between most mild AD individuals and control subjects. These initial results suggest that PET imaging with amyloid tracer may offer the ability to quantitate cerebral amyloid in living humans.

Laboratory testing

Vitamin B$_{12}$ deficiency and hypothyroidism are common co-morbidities in patients with suspected dementia, and screening for these treatable disorders is recommended (Knopman *et al.*, 2001). A few reports have attributed dementia to B$_{12}$ deficiency and hypothyroidism (Clarfield, 1988). In most individuals, treatment of these disorders is unlikely to completely reverse cognitive deficits and cognitive improvement in demented patients with B$_{12}$ and thyroid replacement are equivocal (Knopman *et al.*, 2001). Nevertheless, the high frequency of these co-morbidities and the potential for amelioration of cognitive symptoms necessitates screening (*Table 5.4*). Routine screening for syphilis is no longer recommended, a change from the 1994 practice parameter (AAN, 1994) unless syphilis risk factors or evidence of infection exists.

Table 5.4 Basic laboratory assessment for cognitive impairment

Neuroimaging
- CT
- MRI

Laboratory
- Thyroid
- Vitamin B$_{12}$
- Syphilis (only if clinically indicated)

Pathology of normal brain aging

This topic is covered in considerably more detail in Chapter 4. A brief discussion is presented here as a prelude to discussing the neuropathology of preclinical and overt AD that follows.

A large majority of brains from nondemented persons who show no cognitive impairment at or near the time of death show minimum AD pathology regardless of the age of death. Neocortex sections reveal no, single, or small clusters of isolated a-beta deposits (**5.1**) that are often silver- and thioflavine S-negative or weakly positive. Cerebral amyloid (a-beta) angiopathy (CAA) may or may not be detected. The hippocampal medial CA1 field and entorhinal cortex layer II stellate cells (ERC-II) may show sparse to moderate neurofibrillary tangles (NFTs) that are mostly intra-neuronal. Neuropil threads (NT) are often confined to ERC-II and to transitional allocortex along the descending limb of the collateral sulcus (**5.2**). Braak neurofibrillary staging (Braak & Braak, 1991) (*Box 5.2*, overleaf) is commonly in the stage I–III range. Senile plaques (SP) may be entirely absent from the subcortical regions, basal ganglia, thalamus, brainstem, and cerebellum. Sparse (one or two per section) tangles are often seen in the nucleus basalis of Meynert (NBM), substantia nigra, locus ceruleus, and the dorsal raphe (serotoninergic) nucleus of elderly nondemented (CDR 0) controls (DW McKeel, Jr, personal observation, unpublished) (**5.3**).

5.1 Scattered minute and complex 'satellite' a-beta diffuse plaques with absent neuropil threads or neurofibrillary tangles is the typical histopathologic profile in neocortex sections from autopsied nondemented (CDR 0) persons. (Dual a-beta [red] and PHFtau [black] immunohistochemistry, ×10 objective.)

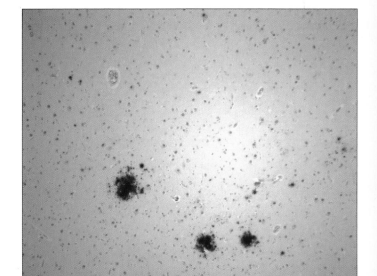

5.2 Cortex of patients with advanced (CDR 3) Alzheimer's disease harbors frequent neuritic senile plaques, neuropil threads, and neurofibrillary tangles. This pattern conforms to Braak stage V/VI (Braak & Braak, 1991). (Dual a-beta [red] and PHFtau [black] immunohistochemistry, ×20 objective.)

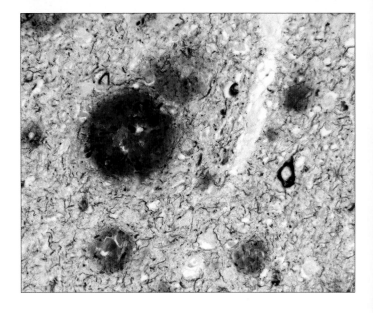

Box 5.2 Gallyas silver staging of neurofibrillary pathology in Alzheimer's disease

The system described by the Braaks (Braak & Braak, 1991) for staging neurofibrillary pathologic lesions in the Alzheimer brain is widely used worldwide. Lesions assessed in medial temporal lobe and occipital neocortex include neurofibrillary tangles, neuropil threads, and neuritic senile plaques. A score is assigned by inspection of silver or tau immunostains on brain tissue sections. Various adaptations of the original methodology have been proposed to increase the practicality of the original method. The method has wide applicability in aging and both pure and mixed forms of AD.

Stage I: Entorhinal cortex neurofibrillary tangles plus neuropil threads

Stage II: Entorhinal cortex (A35) plus hippocampal CA1 neurofibrillary tangles plus neuropil threads

Stage III: A36 lateral to collateral sulcus

Stage IV: Temporal lobe and base of brain

Stage V: Lateral and inferior lateral surface

Stage VI: Entire (holo) cortical neurofibrillary tangles plus neuropil threads

Staging on medial, temporal, and occipital sections

5.3 Incidental globoid neurofibrillary tangles commonly occur in small numbers in locus ceruleus (this image), dorsal raphe nucleus, and nucleus basalis of Meynert in elderly nondemented persons who exhibit no other features of Alzheimer's disease. The brown material is neuromelanin pigment. (H&E, ×40 objective.)

5.4 Widespread argyrophilic diffuse plaques populated the cerebrum (cortex, subcortex, cerebellum, and brainstem) of this 24-year-old nondemented (CDR 0) woman with Down's trisomy 21 syndrome. Microscopic neurofibrillary pathology was entirely absent. (Hedreen-Bielschowsky silver method, ×40 objective.)

Pathology of preclinical AD

During the past 15 years, research in a number of laboratories has indicated that the typical course of AD described above is preceded by a preclinical phase in 20–40% of nondemented individuals (Morris *et al.*, 2004). Insights into this phase of AD include those from carriers of the apolipoprotein E (apoE) epsilon 4 (ε4) allele (Arai *et al.*, 1999), from persons carrying a known mutation in amyloid precursor protein (APP), presenilin 1 (PS1) or presenilin 2 (PS2) genes that cause familial AD (FAD), and from Down's syndrome (DS) patients who carry triple copies of chromosome 21, the source of the APP gene. In DS (trisomy 21), brains from persons who die in their teens and twenties show accumulation of neocortical diffuse SP (**5.4**) in the absence of neurofibrillary pathology such as NFT, NT, and SP dystrophic neurites (DN). DS brains from persons who die in their 30s and early 40s show progressive accumulation of cortical and hippocampal neurofibrillary pathology (Mrak & Griffin, 2004). After age 45, all DS true trisomy cases in the authors' series at the Washington University Alzheimer's Disease Research Center (ADRC)

have typical advanced 'plaque and tangle' AD. Mosaic DS may not be associated with AD pathology at autopsy (Heston, 1984). The dramatic finding of universal histopathology AD in trisomic DS has been confirmed in laboratories throughout the world, thereby providing powerful empirical evidence that accumulation of beta-amyloid, the primary component of SP, drives the neurodegenerative process in AD.

The neuropathology of nonhereditary preclinical AD is characterized by widespread deposition throughout neocortex of preamyloid or diffuse a-beta plaque-like deposits (**5.5**). Neurofibrillary pathology of dorsolateral cortical areas is sparse or absent. Biochemical analyses may demonstrate increases in soluble and total a-beta protein, and in a-beta dimers, that have not yet formed visible SP. CAA may or may not be present. Presence of the apoE ε4 allele enhances the deposition of CAA (Berg *et al.*, 1998). Hippocampal CA1 and ERC-II pyramidal neurons are well preserved in preclinical AD (Price *et al.*, 2001) (**5.6**), although quantitative data in this regard on preclinical AD

5.5 The neocortex of CDR 0.5 cognitively impaired patients with very mild Alzheimer's disease (Morris *et al.*, 1996) and about 25–40% of nondemented CDR 0 persons (Morris *et al.*, 2004; Petersen, 2004) is widely populated by beta amyloid senile plaques (SP). This prefrontal gyrus has SP filling the outer two-thirds, sparing deep cortical layers 5 and 6, and in the immediately subjacent white matter. Neurofibrillary pathology is usually sparse in this circumstance. (A-beta immunostain with brown substrate, ×1 objective.)

5.6 The entorhinal layer II stellate layer neurons are well preserved and free of tangles in many CDR 0 individuals (Price *et al.*, 2001; Roth, 2001). (Modified Bielschowsky silver method, ×10 objective.)

patients who were well characterized during life are meager.

The hippocampus is affected to a mild or moderate degree in preclinical AD. Braak neurofibrillary lesion severity usually is in stages I–IV, with higher stages V and VI being rare (Morris *et al.*, 2004). Brains with predominately or exclusively preamyloid SP, as originally described by Tagliavini (Tagliavini *et al.*, 1988), may exhibit 'hippo-

campal sparing' (**5.7**). The hippocampus contains only a few tangles in medial and lateral CA1 and NTs are absent. Granulovacuolar degeneration (GVD) pathology (**5.8**) is sparse in CA1 neurons. Hirano bodies may be present (**5.9**). In striking contrast in such cases, the neocortex may be filled with a-beta deposits that are thioflavine S- and silver-negative.

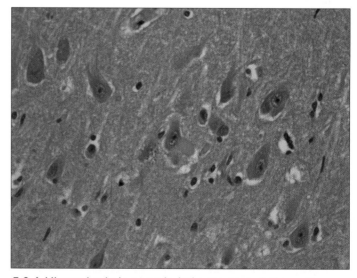

5.7 The hippocampal formation may be spared in a small percentage of persons who have frequent cortical beta amyloid deposits. No senile plaques or neurofibrillary pathology is present. Hippocampal sclerosis, which may account for this 'sparing' pattern, is also absent. (Dual a-beta [red] and PHFtau [black] immunohistochemistry, ×1 objective.)

5.8 The hippocampal CA1 region of AD subjects usually exhibits both accentuated granulovacuolar neuronal degeneration (GVD, black arrow) and Hirano bodies, which are structures composed of paracrystalline lattices of actin (yellow arrow). GVD lesions sequester activated caspase-3 (Cotman & Anderson, 1995) and cytoskeletal components such as tubulin. (H&E, ×60 oil objective.)

5.9 A Hirano body is seen in intimate association with a CA1 hippocampal pyramidal neuron. The bodies by EM are enveloped by neuronal plasma membrane. An adjacent pyramidal neuron exhibits cytoplasmic GVD. (H&E, ×20 objective.)

AD pathology in the preclinical pathologic form of the disease is sparse or absent in other brain regions that are typically heavily affected in more advanced AD. For example, the striatum (caudate and putamen) may contain no or only sparse a-beta deposits (never neuritic SP [NSP]) as may scattered subcortical sites (thalamus, hypothalamus) and the cerebellar cortex. Making a firm and confident criteria-based pathologic diagnosis is difficult in preclinical AD cases. These latter cases would not fulfill standard AD pathologic criteria based on lesion burden in the hippocampus, but amply fulfill the original 1985 National Institute on Aging (NIA) quantitative criteria (Khachaturian, 1985) and modified Washington University ADRC criteria derived from them (McKeel et al., 2004). The Consortium to Establish a Registry for Alzheimer's Disease (CERAD) 1991 criteria (Mirra et al., 1991) that depend exclusively on NSP would not be fulfilled by definition. NIA-Reagan Institute criteria as originally formulated (NIA-Reagan Institute Working Group, 1997) apply only to *demented* cases. Similar pathology occurring in CDR 0.5 AD subjects must be assigned a diagnosis of 'low probability AD' under current NIA-Reagan Institute diagnostic guidelines. The authors' group has proposed that preclinical AD cases be classified in the overall AD spectrum as *very mild preclinical AD* (Morris et al., 2004).

Neuropathology of very mild cognitive impairment (MCI)

Morris et al. in 1991 described the neuropathology of persons who died in the earliest clinically detectable stage of evolving dementia, Clinical Dementia Rating 0.5 (CDR 0.5). The neocortical landscape was strikingly similar to the findings described above in brains from persons with preclinical pathologic AD. In 1996, the authors' group characterized the AD pathology found in 9 of 21 brains from presumed nondemented controls studied longitudinally (Morris et al., 1996). The clinical finding that separated the AD (n=9) versus nonAD pathology (n=12) groups in this second study was a history of at least one CDR 0.5 clinical assessment sometime during the patient's course. The neocortex had widespread and massive deposition of predominately diffuse SP (DSP) that stained well with the Hedreen modification of the Bielschowsky silver method and with antibodies to a-beta. Dual Gallyas silver and a-beta immunostaining showed that 97.3% of prefrontal SP were diffuse (positive for a-beta) and the rest were neuritic as evidenced by their complement of both a-beta and argyrophilic swollen (dystrophic) neurites. Neocortical NFTs and NTs were sparse using both silver and PHFtau immunohistochemistry (IHC). The hippocampal and ERC-II neurofibrillary burden fell in the II–IV Braak staging range (Braak staging was not reported in the paper).

Dr Ronald Peterson's research group at the Mayo Clinic has been instrumental in defining mild cognitive impairment as a clinical entity (Petersen, 2004). They, and others, also recognize that brains of some nondemented persons harbor AD pathology and about 20% of the Mayo series had argyrophilic grain disease (AGD). The authors' nondemented series (Morris et al., 2004) also had a similar high prevalence of AGD (23% of cases with tau-positive and Gallyas-positive limbic grains of Braak; discussed further in Chapter 8) in both the preclinical AD and nonAD groups (see pp. 164–165) (DW McKeel, Jr and JL Price, unpublished data).

Neuropathology of mild, moderate, and severe AD

Overview

As AD progresses across the CDR spectrum, the neocortex undergoes a transformation in which: (1) there is an increasing NSP to DSP ratio, (2) NFTs and NTs progressively accumulate, (3) neurons are lost causing progressive disarray of the cortical laminae, (4) cortical synapses are lost, (5) astrocytic glia undergo hypertrophy and hyperplasia (gliosis), and (6) beta-amyloid species accumulate in meningeal arteries and parenchymal capillaries and arteries (CAA). These changes collectively result in cortical and subcortical atrophy that becomes evident at autopsy. The authors' center uses a visual-based scoring system, which was developed by the Washington University ADRC Neuropathology Core, that allows semi-quantitative scores to be assigned rapidly for both external gyral atrophy and ventricular enlargement seen when the brain is sectioned in the coronal plane (*Box 5.3*, overleaf). Hippocampal and entorhinal temporal lobe atrophy is accompanied by varying degrees of both diffuse and lobar atrophy as AD progresses (*Boxes 5.4, 5.5*) (**5.10A, B**, p. 82).

Box 5.3 Scoring brain atrophy at autopsy: the McKeel–Gado visual-based standards approach

McKeel and Gado in 1994 introduced a new method to score external brain atrophy and ventricular dilatation based on a system of visual standards of formalin-fixed autopsy brains from elderly nondemented and demented subjects. Ventricular scoring was assessed on a 1 to 3+ scale at three rostro-caudal levels of the coronally sectioned cerebrum. External gyral atrophy was based on a panel of external photographs of the lateral portions of the cerebral hemisphere. Scores ranged from normal for age or normal (1+) to moderate (2+) or severe (3+).

Box 5.4 Brain atrophy

Even the healthiest aging is associated with generalized brain atrophy beginning as early as the 4th decade of life and continuing throughout life at annual rate of around 0.4% per year (Fotenos *et al.*, 2005). Brain atrophy likely reflects loss of cortical and subcortical neurons, axonal dropout in the white matter, and shrinkage of large neurons. In these images, age-related brain atrophy is demonstrated by slightly enlarged ventricles and sulcal spaces when comparing axial T1 MRI images (MPRAGE) from a 39-year-old man (**A**) with a nondemented 72-year-old woman (**B**). A number of risk factors in addition to age (Brun & Gustafson, 1976) appear to accelerate the process including hypertension (Gómez-Isla *et al.*, 1996), diabetes (Gómez-Isla *et al.*, 1997), alcohol (Roth, 2001), hyperlipdemia (Cotman & Anderson, 1995), smoking (Horowitz *et al.*, 2004), and homocysteine (Tuszynski *et al.*, 2005).

The presence of AD appears to double the rate of brain atrophy (Brun & Englund, 1981) and pathologic studies suggest cross-sectional and longitudinal estimates of brain atrophy are reflective of neurofibrillary and amyloid plaque burden (Lippa *et al.*, 1992). Accelerated brain atrophy is demonstrated by accentuated sulcal and ventricular spaces in a 75-year-old woman with mild Alzheimer's disease (**C**). In Alzheimer's disease the rate of atrophy is estimated to be about 1% per year. While the presence of brain atrophy is modestly predictive of AD, significant overlap in atrophy pattern between nondemented aging and individuals with AD limit its usefulness in clinical practice as a diagnostic aid.

Box 5.5 Hippocampal atrophy

The hippocampus is an important structure in mediating memory processes (Masliah *et al.*, 2001) and is affected early in AD (Nichols *et al.*, 1995). Hippocampal volume loss is considered a valid biomarker of AD neuropathology (Schechter *et al.*, 1981; Lippa *et al.*, 1992). Magnetic resonance- (MR) based volumetric studies are increasingly being employed as surrogate outcome measures of disease with a particular interest in utilizing hippocampal volume changes as endpoints for measuring AD progression in clinical trials (Onoue *et al.*, 2004). Given inherent test-retest variability of behavioral and cognitive measures, sensitive imaging measures of brain aging may prove important in detecting disease associations, exploring mechanisms of brain aging, and allowing more efficient demonstration of an agent's disease modifying effect.

   Pathological sections obtained at autopsy demonstrate the hippocampus (arrows) and entorhinal cortex (short arrows) in a nondemented individual (**A**) and an individual with late stage AD (**B**). The temporal horn of the ventricle (arrowhead) is greatly enlarged in the demented individual due to severe atrophy of the entorhinal cortex and the hippocampus. Using MRI, the size and shape of hippocampi can be visualized and quantified in life. The hippocampi of a young male (**C**) and an 86-year-old woman with AD (**D**) are outlined in T1-weighted MRI coronal section (red). The hippocampi of the individual with AD is substantially atrophied as demonstrated by the size and the prominence of the temporal ventricular horns. (MRI images courtesy of D Head and RL Buckner.)

5.10 (A) The lateral cerebral hemisphere of an advanced AD patient shows diffuse gyral atrophy with some occipital lobe sparing. **(B)** The brain in **(A)** has been sectioned in the coronal plane at 1 cm intervals. Sulci are gaping and there is marked atrophy of temporal lobe structures including the gray and white matter, amygdala, and hippocampus. The basal ganglia are relatively spared. The temporal horn of the cerebral ventricular system is widely dilated (3+), and the body is moderately (2+) dilated (see *Box 5.5*). Photographs of the fixed brain at autopsy.

Evolution of plaque subtypes

Most authorities would agree that the proportion of total cortical SP that are neuritic increases during the course of AD. Controversy continues, however, on how this occurs. One possibility is that 'amorphous' preamyloid (a-beta nonargyrophilic thioflavine S-negative) SP gradually condense into more compact but still not fully fibrillar diffuse SP. Ordinary light microscopy, especially when differential interference contrast (DIC) optics or silver methods are used, clearly shows linear structures within DSP (**5.11**). The linear theory of SP evolution then holds that DSP acquire dystrophic neurites that stain with silver and hyperphosphorylated tau antibodies to develop into NSP. A small proportion of NSP then develop central compact beta-amyloid protein cores to become cored NSP.

While the foregoing scenario for SP evolution may be true for certain cortical areas, the generalization that *all* SP go through the same evolutionary process may not be accurate. For example, cerebellar a-beta SP may appear compact and stellate, and even have a central dense core (**5.12A, B**), yet they never develop DNs containing abnormal hyperphosphorylated tau (PHFtau). Striatal SP lack associated apoE and remain as DSP throughout the course of AD (Gearing *et al.*, 1997). Medial occipital lobe SP populations have a higher proportion of NSP than DSP at all CDR stages. It is thus clear that local factors in the extracellular tissue milieu, as well as the duration and clinical severity stage of AD, must determine SP morphologic profiles for specific brain regions to a major extent.

Mathematical modeling has been used by several groups to show that SPs are dynamic, porous structures, with SP formation being counterbalanced by SP destruction (Hyman *et al.*, 1993). This is probably mediated by extracellular protease enzymes (Turner *et al.*, 2004). Most recently, Bradley Hyman's group at Harvard Medical School has shown in a series of elegant studies that individual SP tagged with a fluorescent a-beta probe may be observed in a multiphoton microscope over time *in vivo* and their fate can be charted (Christie *et al.*, 2001). Some SP grow (enlarge), some stay the same size over several weeks of observation, and some get smaller in size during the observation period.

5.11 An argyrophilic diffuse senile plaque of a nondemented Down's patient at high optical magnification shows clearly visible internal linear structures that are indicative of a fibrillar substructure. (Modified Bielschowsky method, ×40 objective.)

5.12 Cerebellar beta amyloid deposits may have a streak-like morphology (**A**) or be compact and stellate in shape with a central compact core (**B**). Such 'cored' cerebellar plaques never have any tau-positive internal neuritic staining. (A-beta immunohistochemistry with a brown substrate. **A**: ×10 objective; **B**: ×20 objective.)

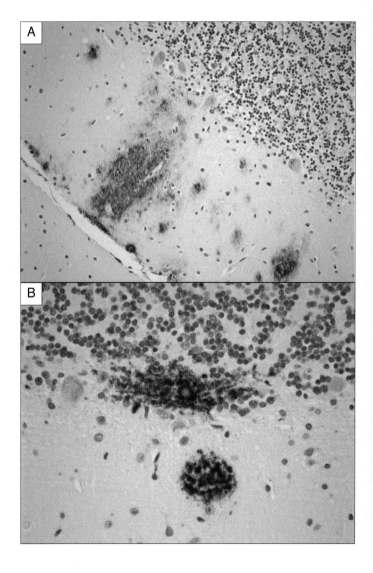

Progression of neurofibrillary pathology

Neurofibrillary pathology (NFP) lesions progressively accumulate, in a hierarchical manner embodied in the Braak staging scheme (Braak & Braak, 1991), in the neocortex of clearly demented AD subjects. Most mild, moderate, and advanced dementia severity AD patients have Braak stage IV–VI brain pathology by the time they die. Perhaps most dramatic is the build-up of aggregated insoluble tau in neuronal processes – axons and dendrites – as NT (**5.13**). At first this process is focal in deeper cortical laminae (V, especially). Cortical layer III then becomes involved so that two 'bands' of tau-positive tangles and NTs appear at low power (**5.14**). Transcortical NT deposition is the rule in persons who die at CDR 3. It is surprising that combined NFP may occupy up to 30% of the cortical ribbon area (DW McKeel, Jr, unpublished observations).

Neuritic plaque PHFtau-positive neurites are a major component of NFP that build up in neocortex in concert with NFT and NT (**5.15A–D**). SP neurites, at various stages of SP evolution, may contain different insoluble protein markers. The a-beta precursor APP is an early marker (Cras *et al.*, 1991), ubiquitin is an intermediate stage marker (He *et al.*, 1993), and PHFtau is a relatively late marker of NSP.

Hippocampal CA1 fields, the subiculum, ERC, and transitional allocortex also accumulate NFT, NT, and NSP during the course of AD (**5.16**). Initially, DSP are progressively replaced by NSP in the outer molecular layer of the dentate fascia, the terminal field of the perforant pathway (**5.17**). Pretangles, best seen in PHFtau or certain silver preparations, harbor granular tau that forms a distinct perinuclear ring (**5.18**). In late stage AD (CDR 3), even the so-called 'silent zone' of the parasubiculum and the clouds of amorphous a-beta protein in the presubiculum accumulate NFT and NT. There is a dramatic replacement of intraneuronal tangles by extracellular ('ghost' or 'tombstone') tangles in both CA1 and ERC-II as AD evolves into the last stages (**5.19**).

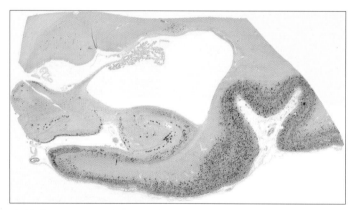

5.13 A typical medial temporal lobe section used for Braak staging of an advanced AD patient brain shows widespread red plaques throughout CA1, dentate fascia, subiculum compartments, entorhinal cortex (ERC), transitional allocortex, and temporal isocortex. Contrasting black neurofibrillary tangles and neuropil threads form a single black band in CA1-subiculum and ERC, then diverge into two distinct bands in allocortex and isocortex. This pattern would be indicative of at least Braak stage IV (Braak & Braak, 1991). Final staging would require examination of the occipital cortex in a preparation such as the one depicted in **5.14** in order to define the total extent of neocortical neurofibrillary pathology. (Dual a-beta [red] and PHFtau [black] immunostain, ×1 objective.)

5.14 PHFtau (PHF-1 tau antibody, gift of Peter Davies) defines two layers of advanced Alzheimer's disease neocortical neurofibrillary pathology. Insoluble tau deposition at this stage (Braak V or VI) is transcortical when viewed at high magnification (see **5.16**). (PHFtau immunohistochemistry with brown substrate, ×1 objective.)

5.15 (A) A neuritic cored senile plaque is surrounded by astrocytes (oval nuclei) and microglia (elongate nuclei). (H&E, ×40 objective.) **(B)** Another cored neuritic plaque stained with modified Bielschowsky silver shows enhanced silver affinity of the compact central amyloid core. (×40 objective.) **(C)** Preamyloid a-beta plaques lack tau neurites but may have central compact amyloid cores (upper right and center plaques). (Dual a-beta [red] and PHFtau [black] immunohistochemistry, 40x objective.) **(D)** A 'mature' cored neuritic plaque contains internal swollen dystrophic neurites that label strongly with PHFtau (black bulbous structures) that contrasts with the red beta amyloid. Note numerous tau-positive neurites at the plaque periphery. (Dual a-beta [red] and PHFtau [black] immunohistochemistry, ×40 objective.)

5.16 (A) Outer entorhinal cortex in advanced AD shows most stellate layer II neurons to have either internal or ghost (extracellular) tau-positive neurofibrillary tangles (larger discreet black structures). Note that some ghost tangles label with a-beta antibody (red substrate), a phenomenon that several laboratories have previously reported. In addition, the entire area is suffused with a myriad of neuropil threads containing aggregated insoluble tau. Numerous red a-beta plaques are evident in the lower cortical laminae. (Dual a-beta [red] and PHFtau [black] immunohistochemistry, ×40 objective.) **(B)** A Gallyas silver preparation of the same brain region shown in panel **(A)** dramatically highlights contorted neuropil threads, tangles and corkscrew-like dendritic processes of entorhinal pyramidal neurons. (Gallyas silver method, ×40 objective.)

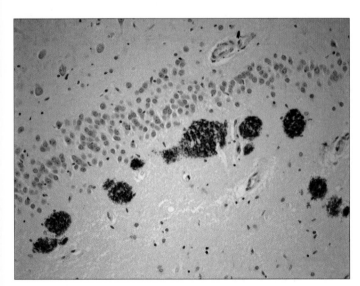

5.17 A row of senile plaques accumulates in advanced AD at the terminal fields of the perforant pathway (PP) within the molecular layer of the dentate fascia of the hippocampal formation. This region is rich in PP synapses that represent the ends of layer II entorhinal cortex stellate neurons. (A-beta amyloid preparation with brown substrate, ×10 objective.)

5.18 Pretangles are an early stage in the development of mature intraneuronal neurofibrillary tangles (NFT). The PHF tau appear more punctate than the condensed fascicles of tau in mature intraneuronal tangles. In addition, there is often a clearly visible perinuclear ring of condensed tau, a so-called 'perinuclear net'. (PHF tau immunohistochemistry, ×40 objective.)

5.19 The Gallyas silver method is excellent for displaying the loose internal structure of ghost tangles that have been partly digested by extracellular proteases. The neuronal cell body has disappeared. Thus, these structures are often referred to as 'tombstone' tangles. They are particularly common in the outer entorhinal cortex (shown here) and in the CA1 region of the hippocampal formation. (Gallyas silver method, ×40 objective.)

Neuronal dysfunction and death

Alterations in neuronal function are undoubtedly a fundamental cause of cognitive impairment and dementia in AD. Functional magnetic resonance imaging (fMRI), MRI spectroscopy, SPECT (single photon emission computed tomography) and positron emission tomography (PET) neuroimaging studies indicate different initial sites of neuronal dysmetabolism (posterior parietal, posterior cingulate) than anatomic studies have generally shown. With but a few previous exceptions (Brun and Gustafson, 1976; Brun and Englund, 1981), more recent histopathologic studies have not shown the initial sites of neuronal and synaptic losses to occur in the posterior parietal and cingulate regions. This striking discrepancy between study modalities needs to be resolved by additional research.

Histopathologic methods including unbiased stereology have shown that certain classes of neurons are lost at different rates during the course of AD. The reasons behind this exquisite *neuronal vulnerability* are surprisingly not well understood. Why, for example, do 60% of ERC-II stellate neurons that give rise to the perforant pathway die by CDR 0.5 (Gómez-Isla *et al.*, 1996)? In contrast, the population of large pyramidal neurons in the superior temporal sulcus are maintained until the late CDR stages (Gómez-Isla *et al.*, 1997).

While the apoptotic cascade has been widely implicated as the primary cause of neuronal death in AD, a substantive body of research indicates that parts of this pathway are bypassed (Cotman & Anderson, 1995; Roth, 2001). Activated caspase-3 has been localized to GVD lesions in hippocampal CA1 pyramidal neurons. Caspase-6 has recently been proposed as a molecular link whereby cytoplasmic subcellular a-beta dimers may trigger changes in tau that lead to paired helical filament and tangle formation (Horowitz *et al.*, 2004). An absolute or relative lack of key growth factors (Tuszynski *et al.*, 2005) or trans-synaptic degeneration may also contribute to selective neuronal death in AD. Together these neuronal death mechanisms combine to cause progressive disarray of the cortical laminae and white matter (axon loss, *Box 5.6*) (**5.20**) at the microscopic level (Brun & Gustafson, 1976; Brun & Englund, 1981).

Box 5.6 White matter lesions

Abnormalities are commonly found in the cerebral white matter in AD and nondemented aging. These white matter lesions (WMLs) are hyperintense on T2 images with corresponding low intensity on T1 images, as seen in an 88-year-old man with mild AD (**A**). For comparison, normal white matter is present in a 76-year-old man with AD (**B**). WMLs are consistently associated with age, hypertension, and other cardiovascular risk factors (Olichney *et al.*, 2000) and are thus commonly considered part of the spectrum of vascular-related injury (Nicoll *et al.*, 2004). In nondemented individuals, WMLs are associated with reduced processing speed, memory, and executive function in nondemented individuals (Nochlin *et al.*, 1998). The clinical significance of WMLs in AD remains less clear. Pathologic studies suggest that individuals with more WMLs have a higher risk of developing AD (Houlden *et al.*, 2000; Bertram & Tanzi, 2004) and require less neuropathologic AD burden to demonstrate cognitive impairment (Lippa *et al.*, 1998) and dementia (Snowdon *et al.*, 1997) than individuals without these lesions. Additionally, radiological studies suggest individuals in the earliest clinical stages of AD may be more vulnerable to the clinically-relevant cognitive influence of WML than nondemented individuals with similar WML burden (Burns *et al.*, 2005).

5.20 Cortical white matter shows severe axon and myelin loss in cases of AD that have remained at CDR 3 for prolonged periods. This modified Bielschowsky silver preparation shows marked axon loss of the deep centrum semiovale in an advanced AD brain. (Modified Bielschowsky silver method, ×40 objective.)

Loss of cortical and hippocampal synapses

The strongest correlation with dementia severity that the authors' research has identified is a correlation of $r^2=0.85$ between CDR at death and the total number of hippocampal synaptophysin-immunoreactive synapses, measured individually by unbiased stereology at ×3,200, in the terminal field of the perforant pathway (NS Havlioglu and DW McKeel, Jr, unpublished data). Approximately 80% of outer molecular layer synapses of the dentate fascia are axon endings of ERC-II stellate neurons (Lippa *et al.*, 1992). Neocortical synapses are also progressively lost during the course of AD. Masliah in collaboration with the authors' group demonstrated loss of prefrontal cortex synaptophysin activity using a dot blot assay in brain homogenates from CDR 0.5 AD individuals (Masliah *et al.*, 2001). Progressive loss of the same marker was shown in the higher CDR groups. Many other laboratories have amply confirmed these findings of profound synaptic loss as a major cause of dementia in general, not just as a key mechanism in AD.

Astrocytic 'gliosis'

Transcription of a major marker of astrocytic glia, the intermediate filament glial fibrillary acidic protein (GFAP), is strongly upregulated during normal aging (Schechter *et al.*, 1981; Nichols *et al.*, 1995). In AD, cortical and hippocampal astrocytes undergo hypertrophy and hyperplasia, a process pathologists refer to as 'gliosis'. Gliosis under the microscope may reflect primarily the enlargement of the astrocyte cell body and processes rather than an actual proliferation of this major glial class (**5.21**). Quantitative image analysis has shown a strong linear and reciprocal increase in cortical glia (primarily astrocytes) at sites where neurons degenerate and are lost (Schechter *et al.*, 1981) (**5.21**).

Cerebral (a-beta) amyloid angiopathy

'Congophilic' amyloid angiopathy was an early name given to this lesion in which beta-pleated sheets of beta-amyloid peptides accumulate in meningeal arteries and parenchymal capillaries and arteries (but rarely in veins) (**5.22A, B**). The dye, Congo red, intercalates into the beta-pleated sheet and exhibits circular dichroism and 'apple green' birefringence under polarized light. Electron microscopy (EM) shows 10 nm twisted filaments. Many proteins as widely diverse as transthyretin and hormones such as glucagon undergo similar physicochemical transformation to form amyloid fibrils *in vivo* or *in vitro* (Onoue *et al.*, 2004). Also, as early as the 1920s, Paul Divry (Attems & Jellinger, 2004) recognized that amyloid proteins may accumulate not only

5.21 The anterior cingulate cortex of an advanced AD patient shows marked neuron loss with replacement gliosis (Brun & Gustafson, 1976; Gómez-Isla *et al.*, 1996; Onoue *et al.*, 2004). The hypertrophied astrocytes have flame-red stellate processes and more cytoplasm than is usually evident in normal brains. (H&E, ×20 objective.)

5.22 (A) Beta amyloid deposition (or formation) is common in the leptomeningeal arterial system in AD. Amyloid-laden blood vessels often have 'double lumens' by H&E. This is a florid example. Note amyloid plaques and tangles in the adjacent brain. (Dual a-beta [red] and PHFtau [black] immunohistochemistry, ×10 objective.) **(B)** Internal and penetrating parenchymal arteries in neocortex may also harbor beta amyloid deposits in AD. (Dual a-beta [red] and PHFtau [black] immunohistochemistry, ×20 objective.)

in arteries but in cerebral capillaries, a lesion he referred to as 'dyshoria'. Divry was apparently struck by the spike-like protrusions extending from the capillary wall into brain parenchyma (**5.23**) and was moved to speculate whether the spikes represented proteinaceous ingress into or egress from the brain. The issue has not been completely settled by recent research.

During the last half of the 20th century three additional methods (described, illustrated, and referenced in Chapter 3) were developed to demonstrate CAA effectively: the Gallyas silver method, thioflavine S and T fluorescent dyes, and immunostaining with a-beta protein antibodies. Although a-beta 1–40 has been identified as a major component of most cases of AD-related CAA, other molecules including a-beta 1–42 and cystatin C may be co-deposited or be the sole cause of CAA (Revesz *et al.*, 2003).

CAA may occur as part of AD or as an isolated lesion in the healthy aging brain. Recent neurosurgical series of operated lobar hemorrhages in elderly persons disclose a high prevalence of CAA that is often thought to be the causative lesion for bleeding (Izumihara *et al.*, 2005). CAA burden in the brain is exacerbated by the presence of one or two apoE e4 alleles (Olichney *et al.*, 2000).

5.23 Capillaries may also become laden with beta-amyloid, especially in medial occipital visual cortex. This example is from entorhinal cortex, a less commonly involved area. Spike-like protrusions of amyloid from brain capillaries have been referred to as 'dyshoric' amyloid angiopathy (e.g. Nicoll *et al.*, 2004; Izumihara *et al.*, 2005). (A-beta immunohistochemistry with brown substrate, ×10 objective.)

The clinically important question is the role that CAA plays in causing or contributing to dementia severity. There is suggestive evidence from series of patients with hereditary CAA syndromes (Dutch, Icelandic, British) that a subset of these patients become demented in the absence of significant AD plaque and tangle pathology (Nicoll *et al.*, 2004). Ultimately this is a difficult question to answer based on current evidence. Assessing mild cognitive impairment and ruling out, for example, preamyloid deposits and early forms of tangles ('pretangles') requires rigorous methodology that has not always been applied to the series mentioned above. Although admittedly subject to challenge, it is the author's belief that CAA can cause progressive cognitive impairment as the sole or dominant dementing pathology.

Comparing sporadic and familial AD

The pathology of DS trisomy 21, a form of genetically determined dementia, has already been described in this chapter. Similar to many pedigrees with a mutation in APP, PS1 or PS2, DS cerebral pathology and dementia appear decades before similar clinical and pathologic changes do in brains of sporadic AD patients. Some PS1 mutations (Nochlin *et al.*, 1998) lead to unusually severe CAA. 'Cotton wool plaques' are another lesion that has been recently described in brains of persons with PS1 mutations (Houlden *et al.*, 2000). A worldwide intensive search is underway to define additional risk factors besides the apoE ε4 allele and APP or presenilin gene mutations that determine the variable age of onset in very early onset (before age 40), early onset (before age 65) and late onset sporadic and FAD (Bertram & Tanzi, 2004).

Another intriguing aspect of FAD pathology is the higher than expected prevalence of co-occurring Lewy body disease. Lippa *et al.* (1998), for example, found that a majority of FAD brains harbored Lewy bodies demonstrable with alpha-synuclein immunohistochemistry (IHC) in the amygdala. The authors have studied a small pedigree in which three members from two generations had autosomal dominant AD with onset in their 20s and death 10–20 years later. One brain from a 43-year-old affected woman who survived 19 years weighed only 700 g and exhibited global knife edge gyral atrophy and severe diffuse ventricular enlargement (**5.24A, B**) at autopsy. The neocortex and hippocampus showed typical severe AD plaque and tangle with CAA pathology (**5.25**).

5.24 (**A**) A lateral view of the formalin-fixed 700 g brain at autopsy from a 43-year-old woman with familial AD who survived 19 years. Note the striking overall size decrease of the cerebrum compared to the cerebellum. Also noted the marked sulcal narrowing that involves all four major lobes and approaches a 'knife-edge' appearance focally. (**B**) The same brain after being sectioned at 1 cm intervals in the coronal plane. All portions are severely affected including the deep white matter, basal ganglia, and hippocampal formation. Autopsy fixed brain specimen.

5.25 Microscopically, the brain shown in **5.24** and **5.26** revealed florid deposition of beta-amyloid and the full extent of tau-positive neurofibrillary pathology. This section of the subicular complex has numerous confluent amyloid plaques (red) and tangles (black). (Dual a-beta [red] and PHFtau [black] immunohistochemistry, ×20 objective.)

Abundant Lewy pathology in the form of classical Lewy bodies (substantia nigra), Lewy neurites that occurred diffusely and concentrated in the hippocampal CA1/2 (sometimes referred to as CA2/3) junction, and cortical Lewy bodies, was detected throughout brainstem, limbic structures (including the amygdala), and neocortical areas using alpha-synuclein IHC (**5.26A**, **B**). Additional information about the co-occurrence of AD and Lewy pathology is presented in Chapter 7.

5.26 (**A**) The mid-brain substantia nigra of the familial AD case depicted in **5.24** and **5.25** also showed classical Lewy bodies. Note the basophilic darker center and the clear halo that separates the filamentous inclusion from the surrounding cell cytoplasm. Oligodendrocytes and a small arteriole with red blood cells (7 μm diameter) in the lumen may be used for size comparisons). (H&E stain, ×40 objective.) (**B**) The same brain also revealed widespread limbic (not shown) and neocortical Lewy bodies (CLBs). Four clustered CLBs in superior temporal cortex are strongly labeled with alpha-synuclein (aSYN) antibody LB-509. Lewy neurites that are also aSYN positive are present in the adjacent neuropil. (Alpha synuclein immunohistochemistry, ×40 objective.)

References

American Academy of Neurology/Quality Standards Subcommittee (1994). Practice parameter for diagnosis and evaluation of dementia. *Neurology* **44**:2203–2206.

Arai T, Ikeda K, Akiyama H, *et al.* (1999). A high incidence of apolipoprotein E epsilon 4 allele in middle-aged non-demented subjects with cerebral amyloid beta protein deposits. *Acta Neuropathol.* **97**(1):82–84.

Attems J, Jellinger KA (2004). Only cerebral capillary amyloid angiopathy correlates with Alzheimer pathology – a pilot study. *Acta Neuropathol.* **107**(2):83–90.

Berg L, McKeel DW Jr, Miller JP, *et al.* (1998). Clinicopathologic studies in cognitively healthy aging and Alzheimer disease: relation of histologic markers to dementia severity, age, sex, and apolipoprotein E genotype. *Arch. Neurol.* **55**(3):326–335.

Bertram L, Tanzi RE (2004). The current status of Alzheimer's disease genetics: what do we tell the patients? (Review) (83 refs). *Pharmacol. Res.* **50**(4):385–396.

Braak H, Braak E (1991). The neuropathologic stageing of Alzheimer-related changes. *Acta Neuropathol. (Berlin)* **82**:239–259.

Brun A, Englund E (1976). Regional pattern of degeneration in Alzheimer's disease: neuronal loss and histopathological grading. *Histopathology* **5**:459–464.

Brun A, Gustafson L (1976). Distribution of cerebral degeneration in Alzheimer's disease. A clinico-pathological study. *Archiv fur Psychiatrie und Nervenkrankheiten* **223**(1):15–33.

Burns JM, Church JA, Johnson DK, *et al.* (2005). White matter lesions are prevalent but differentially related with cognition in aging and early Alzheimer's disease. *Arch. Neurol.* **62**:1870–1876.

Christie RH, Bacskai BJ, Zipfel WR, *et al.* (2001). Growth arrest of individual senile plaques in a model of Alzheimer's disease observed by *in vivo* multiphoton microscopy. *J. Neurosci.* 21(3):858–864.

Chui H, Zhang Q (1997). Evaluation of dementia: a systematic study of the usefulness of the American Academy of Neurology's practice parameters. *Neurology* 49:925–935.

Clarfield AM (1988). The reversible dementias: do they reverse? *Ann. Intern. Med.* 109:476–486.

Cotman CW, Anderson AJ (1995). A potential role for apoptosis in neurodegeneration and Alzheimer's disease. *Mol. Neurobiol.* 10:19–45.

Cras P, Kawai M, Lowery D, *et al.* (1991). Senile plaque neurites in Alzheimer disease accumulate amyloid precursor protein. *Proc. Nat. Acad. Sci. USA* 88(17):7552–7556.

Ebly EM, Parhad IM, Hogan DB, *et al.* (1994). Prevalence and types of dementia in the very old: results from the Canadian Study of Health and Aging. *Neurology* 44(9):1593–1600.

Fotenos AF, Snyder AZ, Girton LE, *et al.* (2005). Normative estimates of cross-sectional and longitudinal brain volume decline in aging and AD. *Neurology* 64:1032–1039.

Gearing M, Levey AI, Mirra SS (1997). Diffuse plaques in the striatum in Alzheimer disease (AD): relationship to the striatal mosaic and selected neuropeptide markers. *J. Neuropathol. Exp. Neurol.* 56:1363–1370.

Gómez-Isla T, Hollister R, West H, *et al.* (1997). Neuronal loss correlates with but exceeds neurofibrillary tangles in Alzheimer's disease. *Ann. Neurol.* 41:17–24.

Gómez-Isla T, Price JL, McKeel DW Jr, *et al.* (1996). Profound loss of layer II entorhinal cortex neurons in very mild Alzheimer's disease. *J. Neurosci.* 16:4491–4500.

He Y, Delaere P, Duyckaerts C, *et al.* (1993). Two distinct ubiquitin immunoreactive senile plaques in Alzheimer's disease: relationship with the intellectual status in 29 cases. *Acta Neuropathol.* 86(1):109–116.

Hebert LE, Beckett LA, Scherr PA, *et al.* (2001). Annual incidence of Alzheimer disease in the United States projected to the years 2000 through 2050. *Alz. Dis. Assoc. Dis.* 15(4):169–173.

Heston LL (1984). Down's syndrome and Alzheimer's dementia: defining an association. (Review) (15 refs) *Psych. Develop.* 2:287–294.

Horowitz PM, Patterson KR, Guillozet-Bongaarts AL, *et al.* (2004). Early N-terminal changes and caspase-6 cleavage of tau in Alzheimer's disease. *J. Neurosci.* 24(36):7895–7902.

Houlden H, Baker M, McGowan E, *et al.* (2000). Variant Alzheimer's disease with spastic paraparesis and cotton wool plaques is caused by PS1 mutations that lead to exceptionally high amyloid-b concentrations. *Ann. Neurol.* 48:806–808.

Hyman BT, Marzloff K, Arriagada PV (1993). The lack of accumulation of senile plaques or amyloid burden in Alzheimer's disease suggests a dynamic balance between amyloid deposition and resolution. *J. Neuropathol. Exp. Neurol.* 52(6):594–600.

Izumihara A, Suzuki M, Ishihara T (2005). Recurrence and extension of lobar hemorrhage related to cerebral amyloid angiopathy: multivariate analysis of clinical risk factors. *Surg. Neurol.* 64(2):160–164.

Khachaturian ZS (1985). Diagnosis of Alzheimer's disease. *Arch. Neurol.* 42:1097–1105.

Knopman DS, DeKosky ST, Cummings JL, *et al.* (2001). Practice parameter: diagnosis of dementia (an evidence-based review). Report of the Quality Standards Subcommittee of the American Academy of Neurology. *Neurology* 56:1143–1153.

Lippa CF, Fujiwara H, Mann DM, *et al.* (1998). Lewy bodies contain altered alpha-synuclein in brains of many familial Alzheimer's disease patients with mutations in presenilin and amyloid precursor protein genes. *Am. J. Pathol.* 153(5):1365–1370.

Lippa CF, Hamos JE, Pulaski-Salo D, *et al.* (1992). Alzheimer's disease and aging: effects on perforant pathway perikarya and synapses. *Neurobiol. Aging* 13(3):405–411.

Masliah E, Mallory M, Alford M, *et al.* (2001). Altered expression of synaptic proteins occurs early during progression of Alzheimer's disease. *Neurology* 56:127–129.

McKeel DW Jr, Price JL, Miller JP, *et al.* (2004). Neuropathologic criteria for diagnosing Alzheimer Disease in persons with pure dementia of Alzheimer type. *J. Neuropathol. Exp. Neurol.* 63:1028–1037.

McKhann G, Drachman D, Folstein M, *et al.* (1984). Clinical diagnosis of Alzheimer's disease: report of the NINCDS-ADRDA Work Group under the auspices of Department of Health and Human Services Task Force on Alzheimer's disease. *Neurology* 34:939–944.

Mendez MF, Cummings JL (2003). Alzheimer's Disease. In: *Dementia: A Clinical Approach*. 3rd edn. Butterworth Heinemann, Philadelphia, pp. 67–95.

Mintun MA, LaRossa GN, Sheline YI, *et al.* (2006). ["C]PIB in a nondemented polulation: potential antecedent marker of Alzheimer's disease. *Neurology* 67:446–452.

Mirra SS, Heyman A, McKeel D Jr, *et al.* (1991). The Consortium to Establish a Registry for Alzheimer's Disease (CERAD). Part II. Standardization of the neuropathologic assessment of Alzheimer's disease. *Neurology* **41**:479–486.

Morris JC, McKeel DW Jr, Buckles VD, *et al.* (2004). Neuropathological markers of preclinical Alzheimer's disease in nondemented aging. *J. Neurosci. Abstr.* **902** online (URL: http://sfn.scholarone.com/itin2004/index.html).

Morris JC, McKeel DW Jr, Storandt M, *et al.* (1991). Very mild Alzheimer's disease: informant-based clinical, psychometric, and pathological distinction from normal aging. *Neurology* **41**:469–478.

Morris JC, Storandt M, McKeel DW Jr, *et al.* (1996). Cerebral amyloid deposition and diffuse plaques in 'normal' aging: evidence for presymptomatic and very mild Alzheimer's disease. *Neurology* **46**:707–729.

Mrak RE, Griffin WS (2004). Trisomy 21 and the brain. (Review) (78 refs) *J. Neuropathol. Exp. Neurol.* **63**(7):679–685.

NIA-Reagan Institute Working Group consensus recommendations for the postmortem diagnosis of Alzheimer's disease (1997). The National Institute on Aging, and Reagan Institute Working Group on Diagnostic Criteria for Neuropathological Assessment of Alzheimer's disease. *Neurobiol. Aging* **18**(4 Suppl):S1–S2.

Nichols NR, Finch CE, Nelson JF (1995). Food restriction delays the age-related increase in GFAP mRNA in rat hypothalamus. *Neurobiol. Aging* **16**(1):105–110.

Nicoll JA, Yamada M, Frackowiak J, *et al.* (2004). Cerebral amyloid angiopathy plays a direct role in the pathogenesis of Alzheimer's disease. Pro-CAA position statement. (Review) (61 refs). *Neurobiol. Aging* **25**(5):589–597; discussion 603–604.

Nochlin D, Bird TD, Nemens EJ, *et al.* (1998). Amyloid angiopathy in a Volga German family with Alzheimer's disease and a presenilin-2 mutation (N141I). (Case Reports.) *Ann. Neurol.* **43**:131–135.

Olichney JM, Hansen LA, Lee JH, *et al.* (2000). Relationship between severe amyloid angiopathy, apolipoprotein E genotype, and vascular lesions in Alzheimer's disease. (Review) (31 refs). *Annals NY Acad. Sci.* **903**:138–143.

Onoue S, Ohshima K, Debari K, *et al.* (2004). Mishandling of the therapeutic peptide glucagon generates cytotoxic amyloidogenic fibrils. *Pharm. Res.* **21**(7):1274–1283.

Petersen RC (2004). Mild cognitive impairment as a diagnostic entity. (Review) (50 refs) *J. Int. Med.* **256**(3):183–194.

Price JL, Ko AI, Wade MJ, *et al.* (2001). Neuron number in entorhinal cortex and CA1 in preclinical Alzheimer's disease. *Arch. Neurol.* **58**:1395–1402.

Reisberg B, Ferris SH, de Leon MJ, *et al.* (1982). Global Deterioration Scale. *Am. J. Psych.* **139**:1136–1139.

Revesz T, Ghiso J, Lashley T, *et al.* (2003). Cerebral amyloid angiopathies: a pathologic, biochemical, and genetic view. (Review) (80 refs). *J. Neuropathol. Exp. Neurol.* **62**:885–898.

Roth KA (2001). Caspases, apoptosis, and Alzheimer disease: causation, correlation, and confusion. (Review) (84 refs). *J. Neuropathol. Exp. Neurol.* **60**(9):829–838.

Sano M (2004). A guide to diagnosis of Alzheimer's disease. *CNS Spectrums* **9**(7 Suppl 5):16–19.

Schechter R, Yen SH, Terry RD (1981). Fibrous astrocytes in senile dementia of the Alzheimer type. *J. Neuropathol. Exp. Neurol.* **40**(2):95–101.

Small GW, Rabins PV, Barry PP, *et al.* (1997). Diagnosis and treatment of Alzheimer disease and related disorders. Consensus statement of the American Association for Geriatric Psychiatry, the Alzheimer's Association, and the American Geriatrics Society. *JAMA* **278**:1363–1371.

Snowdon DA, Greiner LH, Mortimer JA, *et al.* (1997). Brain infarction and the clinical expression of Alzheimer disease. *JAMA* **277**:813–817.

Tagliavini F, Giaccone G, Frangione B, *et al.* (1988). Preamyloid deposits in the cerebral cortex of patients with Alzheimer's disease and nondemented individuals. *Neurosci. Lett.* **93**(2–3):191–196.

Turner AJ, Fisk L, Nalivaeva NN (2004). Targeting amyloid-degrading enzymes as therapeutic strategies in neurodegeneration. *Ann. NY Acad. Sci.* **1035**:1–20.

Tuszynski MH, Thal L, Pay M, *et al.* (2005). A phase 1 clinical trial of nerve growth factor gene therapy for Alzheimer disease. *Nature Medicine* **11**(5):551–555.

Chapter 6

Neuropathology of vascular dementia

Introduction

Vascular dementia (VaD) refers to cognitive impairment resulting from cerebrovascular disease and ischemic brain injury, such as infarcts and leukoaraiosis. Although prevalence estimates are quite variable, VaD is considered by many to be the second most common cause of dementia, accounting for 10–25% (Fratiglioni et al., 2000; Jellinger, 2002a) of cases of dementia. The diagnosis of VaD, however, has been problematic largely related to the absence of consensus criteria for both the pathologic and clinical diagnosis of the disorder.

Clinical features

The clinical course of VaD is often marked by an abrupt onset with stepwise progression (periods of stability followed by sudden decrements in function). Physical examination often reveals corticospinal or corticobulbar signs (increased reflexes, Babinski's sign, gait abnormalities, weakness). Computed tomography (CT) and magnetic resonance imaging (MRI) studies reveal variable findings, including cortical infarcts in the territory of a major artery (**6.1**), lacunar infarcts less than 1.5 cm in diameter (**6.2**), and white matter (WM) lesions marked by abnormal signal intensity (**6.3**). VaD patients are more likely to have relative preservation of long-term memory, with greater deficits in frontal executive functioning compared with Alzheimer's disease (AD) patients. The neuropsychological hallmark of vascular dementia is generally considered to be frontal executive dysfunction related to interruption of frontal–subcortical circuits.

Cardinal features

Cardinal features in the clinical criteria for VaD include: (1) the presence of a dementia syndrome with (2) objective documentation of vascular lesions capable of causing dementia. These two critical elements in the criteria are variably defined across different VaD criteria (*Tables 6.1, 6.2*) (Verhey et al., 1996). Since the 1970s, several clinical criteria for VaD have been developed. The most widely used vascular dementia criteria in clinical studies is the

---

Table 6.1 Clinical criteria for vascular dementia

- Diagnostic and Statistical Manual of Mental Disorders, Fourth Edition (DSM-IV) (APA, 1994)
- International Classification of Diseases, Tenth Revision (ICD-10) (WHO, 1993)
- California Alzheimer's Disease Diagnostic and Treatment Center criteria (ADDTC) (Chui et al., 1992)
- National Institute of Neurologic Disorders and Stroke – Association Internationale pour la Recherche et L'Enseignement En Neurosciences criteria (NINDS-AIREN) (Roman et al., 1993)
- CCCCCR (Canadian Consortium) (Rockwood et al., 1994)
- Hachinski Ischemic Score (Rosen et al., 1980)

6.1 T1 and T2 images from a 67-year-old man who presented with 2 months of speech disturbance ('mumbling', halting speech), difficulty with language comprehension (described as 'hard of hearing'), and right-sided clumsiness. T2-weighted images (proton density, images **A–D**) reveal extensive encephalomalacia throughout the left middle cerebral artery territory. There is compensatory dilation of the left ventricle and cortical atrophy, best visualized on the T1 images (images **E–H**). Carotid ultrasound revealed complete occlusion of the left internal carotid artery. Collateral sources of blood flow to regions of the cortex are likely to have allowed sparing of some regions of the cortex, with most damage apparent in the subcortical regions. Improvement was noted over the ensuing months but chronic deficits persisted in speech (anomia, nonfluent speech) in addition to mild right-hand weakness and sensory impairment.

6.2 This 75-year-old African American male had a progressive, gradual decline in cognition that began at the age of 69 with symptoms including difficulty driving, misplacing items, and reduced judgment and problem solving. His symptoms progressed gradually in the ensuing 8 years. His medical history was notable during this time for the occurrence of several transient ischemic attacks. MRI 2 weeks before death for fever and unresponsiveness revealed significant white matter changes and an infarct in the left thalamus (arrow). At the time of death from sepsis and cachexia, he was judged to have severe Alzheimer's dementia

with cerebrovascular disease (CDR 3). Neuropathological examination revealed the absence of amyloid plaques and tangles in the cortex and multiple infarcts in the basal ganglia and white matter.

6.3 MRI images (FLAIR) (**A**, **B**) demonstrating white matter lesions as defined by high signal abnormalities. White matter lesions are considered part of the spectrum of vascular-related injury (Bernick *et al.*, 2001), due to their consistent association with hypertension and cardiovascular risk factors (Longstreth *et al.*, 1996). T1 (**C**) and T2 (**D**) images demonstrating periventricular white matter lesions (arrow), deep white matter lesions (curved arrow), and an infarct in the left caudate (open arrow). While white matter lesions are high signal on T2 and FLAIR images, they have corresponding low intensity signal on T1 images. Infarcts have similar intensities as cerebrospinal fluid and thus are darker on T1 and brighter on T2 images than white matter lesions.

Table 6.2 American Psychiatric Association DSM-IV definition for vascular dementia

- Cognitive deficits resulting in significant impairment in social or occupational functioning representing a decline from higher level of functioning
- Focal neurological signs, symptoms and imaging evidence are judged to be etiologically related to the cognitive disturbance
- The course is characterized by sustained periods of clinical stability, punctuated by sudden significant cognitive and functional losses
- Deficits do not occur in the course of delirium exclusively

(APA, 1994)

NINDS–AIREN research criteria (Roman *et al.*, 1993), which operationalizes probable VaD as the presence of dementia, evidence of cerebrovascular disease, and a clear temporal relationship between the two (*Table 6.3*). The modified Hachinski Ischemic Score (Rosen *et al.*, 1980) (*Table 6.4*) may be useful in identifying the majority of dementia patients with at least some cerebrovascular pathology (del Ser *et al.*, 1990; Knopman *et al.*, 2001).

Diagnostic difficulties

There is significant clinical variability in the presentation of VaD, with up to 50% of cases having an insidious onset and progressive course while only 34% have an abrupt onset with stepwise progression. This makes the recognition of pure VaD difficult. The choice of criteria employed in diagnosing VaD clinically leads to large variability in prevalence estimates, identification of different groups of subjects, and differences in the type and distribution of brain lesions. The Cardiovascular Health Study (CHS) classified 3600 CHS participants using various clinical criteria (Lopez *et al.*, 2005). The investigators found that none of the clinical criteria for VaD identified the same group of subjects and differentiating VaD from AD was difficult.

The boundaries defining AD and VaD remain unclearly defined. Of AD cases, 40% have mixed pathologies, most commonly cerebrovascular disease, while pure cases of VaD are rare. A survey of 1929 autopsied cases of dementia found only six with a pure VaD (Hulette *et al.*, 1997). Most neuropathologic studies of VaD reveal the unexpected presence of AD with or without concomitant strokes (Berg *et al.*, 1998; Longstreth *et al.*, 1996; Bernick *et al.*, 2001). The few clinicopathologic studies of mixed dementia indicate that cerebrovascular lesions have an important role in contributing to AD onset and severity (Heyman *et al.*, 1998; Jellinger *et al.*, 2003; de la Torre, 2004). Thus, VaD appears to be both underdiagnosed (Korczyn, 2005) and overdiagnosed (Brust, 1983) clinically, at least in the US.

These problems highlight the need for further studies to refine the diagnostic criteria and the identification of different categories of this disorder. This heterogeneity in the clinical characterization of the disorder is compounded by the lack of consensus regarding the pathologic diagnosis of VaD. Unfortunately, the clinical and pathologic concept of the disorder has not yet found a simple translation into clinical practice.

Table 6.3 NINDS-AIREN criteria for probable vascular dementia

- Dementia
- Evidence of cerebrovascular disease (focal signs on exam and relevant imaging findings including multiple large vessel strokes or a single strategically placed infarct)
- Temporal relationship between dementia and cerebrovascular disease: onset of dementia within 3 months following recognized stroke, or an abrupt deterioration in cognitive functions, or fluctuating stepwise progression of cognitive deficits
- Supportive features: gait disturbance, history of unsteadiness or unprovoked falls, early urinary frequency, and personality and mood changes including depression, abnormal executive function, and psychomotor retardation

(Roman *et al.*, 1993)

Table 6.4 Modified Hachinski Score

Feature	Value
Abrupt onset	2
Fluctuating course	2
History of strokes	2
Focal neurologic signs	2
Focal neurologic symptoms	2
Stepwise deterioration	1
Nocturnal confusion	1
Relative preservation of personality	1
Depression	1
Somatic complaints	1
Emotional incontinence	1
Hypertension	1
Evidence of atherosclerosis	1

(Hachinski *et al.*, 1975; Rosen *et al.*, 1980)

Box 6.1 A simplified clinical–neuropsychological comparison of vascular dementia (VaD) with Alzheimer's disease (AD) at the mild–moderate stage

Clinical profile:	VaD	AD
Prevalence among dementias	15%	70%
Common presenting complaints	Abrupt change in cognitive/physical performance, reduced cognitive flexibility, verbal retrieval deficit	Forgetfulness
Neurological/motor	Risk and/or history of cerebrovascular disease, gait disturbance	Normal functioning
Neuropsychiatric	Depression, apathy, agitation	Depression, anxiety, delusions
Course from diagnosis to death	Varies widely (5–15 years)	8–10 years
Progression	Stepwise decline with fluctuation	Gradual downward decline

Neuropsychological profile:		
Qualitative performance differences	Fluctuating cognition, perseverative errors, variable self-monitoring, performance benefits from verbal cueing	Forgetfulness for instructions, receptive language problems
Confusion/disorientation	++	+
Attention/concentration deficits	+++	++
Episodic memory deficits	++	++++
Language deficits	+++	++
Executive dysfunction	+++	+++
Visual–spatial deficits	+	+
ADL impairment	++	++

Studies comparing the neuropsychology of VaD variants and AD are not consistent with regards to differences and point to significant overlap in clinical presentations. The table above emphasizes differences suggested by a relatively greater subcortical involvement. Based on published findings and clinical criteria, + signs estimate relative impairment in a given cognitive-functional domain when assessed at the mild to moderate stage of disease progression. Fewer + signs indicate less impaired functioning. Vascular lesions will impact cognition and function in various ways depending on lesion type, number, size, distribution, and progression over time. VaD subtypes include multi-infarct dementia (where involvement of cortical vs. subcortical regions may show different deficit profiles), strategic single-infarct dementia, small vessel disease dementia, hypoperfusion, hemorrhagic dementia, and various mixed etiologies. Approximately 25% of persons with AD, for example, also have vascular changes which may further exacerbate deficits. It is important to recognize that clinical presentations of these disorders will vary across individuals, especially when mixed dementia pathologies are present.

(McPherson & Cummings, 1996; Desmond, 2004; Garrett et al., 2004; Graham et al., 2004; Sachdev et al., 2004.)

The role of psychological tests in diagnosing VaD

Neuropsychological profiles of AD and VaD patients may differ in some tests but may not be sufficient by themselves to discriminate reliably between the two conditions (Loring *et al.*, 1986; Lindeboom *et al.*, 2004). Loring *et al.* (1986) found that VaD and AD research subjects differed in three specific tests: FSIQ (Wechsler Adult Intelligence Scale (WAIS) – Revised Full Scale IQ), VIQ (WAIS – Verbal IQ), and Picture Completion. This contrasted to no difference in verbal memory, visual–spatial skills, and sustained attention/concentration. They concluded: 'neuro-psychological testing of elderly patients is unable to aid in the differential diagnosis between similar forms of dementia.'

Clinical risk factors

Interestingly, AD and cerebrovascular disease show common risk factors including hypertension, hyper-cholesterolemia, diabetes, apolipoprotein E (Roman, 2004). Some have suggested that the pathophysiology of AD and cerebrovascular disease may be etiologically linked. Others have found that infarcts may precipitate dementia through an additive or synergistic relationship with AD neuropathology. Nonetheless, an emerging picture is that mixed dementia may be the most common form of dementia (AD with cerebrovascular disease).

Treatment

A full discussion of the treatment of cerebrovascular disease as related to VaD is beyond the scope of this atlas. Randomized controlled trials of cholinesterase inhibitors have been conducted in VaD and mixed dementia and have shown a similar magnitude of benefit as observed in AD. Thus, traditional AD therapy is likely to be of modest benefit in VaD. Additionally, cerebrovascular disease is known to be preventable. While randomized controlled trials remain absent, it is hoped that aggressive treatment of cerebrovascular risk factors in middle age may reduce the incidence of dementia and AD. Epidemiologic studies suggest a decreased incidence of cognitive decline in those aggressively treated with antihypertensives, cholesterol lowering agents, and aspirin.

Neuropathology of VaD

Prevalence and incidence of vascular dementia

Although VaD is said to be the second or third most common form of dementia in some series (Fratiglioni *et al.*, 2000; Jellinger, 2002a; Ikeda *et al.*, 2004), studies conducted in North American academic centers indicate that VaD rarely exists as the sole dementing pathology (Nolan *et al.*, 1998). The latter study and others (Hulette *et al.*, 1997) suggest that isolated pure VaD is rare as a pure clinicopathologic entity. Studies that indicate VaD is the second most common form of dementia, accounting for up to 25% of all cases in adults, usually lack autopsy confirmation to demonstrate that AD or related neurodegenerative lesions are not co-occurring disorders.

The pathologist's dilemma in diagnosing VaD

The pathologist faces several difficulties in making a confident diagnosis of VaD: (1) validated pathologic criteria for pure VaD do not exist; (2) small vascular lesions such as microinfarcts, microaneurysms, and segmental arteriosclerosis are common lesions in the nondemented elderly (refer to Chapter 4); (3) complex interactions between competing risk factors are often not known or considered; and (4) comprehensive unbiased pathological mapping of the many varieties of cerebral vascular disease is daunting.

Diagnostic criteria for VaD

A number of clinical diagnostic criteria for VaD have been published using various combinations of the pathologic features enumerated in this chapter (Chui *et al.*, 1992; WHO, 1992, 1993; Roman *et al.*, 1993; APA, 1994; Chui *et al.*, 2000). Most investigators would agree that none of these criteria have the required sensitivity and specificity to identify patients reliably with mixed VaD. The Hachinski scale/score (Rosen *et al.*, 1980) has been validated by autopsy studies (Fischer *et al.*, 1991; Moroney *et al.*, 1997a,b), showing that serious VaD can be screened for by this simple measure alone. However, milder vascular pathology can only be detected reliably using imaging technology. Unfortunately, imaging data targeted at defining vascular pathology are frequently not available for dementia patients, and are therefore lacking in many published series of AD, Lewy body, and frontotemporal dementia (FTD) patients.

Risk factors that influence VaD pathology

Intensive efforts are currently being focused on vascular factors that contribute to many dementing disorders as well as preclinical and mild cognitive impairments that precede overt dementia. The reason is that many of these vascular components are amenable to existing therapeutic interventions (*Table 6.5*).

Characteristic pathologic lesions of VaD

Table 6.6 lists the main VaD lesions that will be considered in this chapter. The lesion categories are those referenced in the NACC (National Alzheimer Coordinating Center, Seattle WA) *Neuropathology Manual*, version 2.0.

Atherosclerosis

Risk factors such as age, cholesterol and lipid metabolism, diabetes mellitus, hypertension, the apoE ε4 allele, male gender, dietary intake, obesity, level of exercise and many other factors interact similarly with the cerebral vasculature as they do with systemic arterial vascular beds (heart, kidney) to modulate the pathologic expression of atherosclerosis (AS) (Moossy, 1993). These factors tend to increase severity of AS but protective factors exist as well.

AS affects the larger blood vessels of the cerebral circulation: aortic arch, carotid and vertebral arteries, the arterial Circle of Willis (COW) (**6.4**), and meningeal and parenchymal arteries including the medullary penetrating

---

Table 6.5 Treatable vascular lesions that may contribute to mild cognitive deficits and to overt dementia

Vascular lesion/disorder	Treatment/intervention
Atherosclerosis, especially of the aortic arch	Statins (lower cholesterol); antiplatelet therapy
Hypertension	Antihypertensive regimen to lower systolic and diastolic blood pressure (beta-blockers, calcium channel blockers, diuretics, diet and life style adjustments)
Diabetic microangiopathy and microaneurysms	Insulin, oral hyperglycemics to bring fasting blood sugar into normal range
Cerebral infarction	Early: tissue plasminogen activator to dissolve thrombi Late: treatment to improve blood flow to ischemic 'penumbra' Antiplatelet and aspirin for transient ischemic attack prophylaxis
Cerebral hemorrhage	Antihypertensives
Cerebral amyloid angiopathy	Presence of notch gene mutation Establish apoE genotype and presence or absence of ε4 alleles
Cerebral aneurysm	Angiographic localization followed by ligation, surgical embolism to cause thrombosis
Multi-infarct dementia	Control systemic and cerebral vascular risk factors
CADASIL	Recognize notch-3 gene mutation and treat as high-risk infarct or hemorrhage-prone patient
Critical CAD (≥75% narrowing)	By-pass, stenting, reduce cardiovascular risk factors, statins, anti-platelet therapy
Carotid stenosis	Endarterectomy surgery; arterial bypass surgery
Hyperlipidemia, hereditary	Statins, life style change with diet
Inherited clotting factor defects	Diagnosis; bleeding diathesis

(CAD: cerebral artery disease; CADASIL: cerebral autosomal dominant arteriopathy with subcortical infarcts and leukoencephalopathy)

Table 6.6 Pathologic basis for vascular dementia

Lesion	Common locations
Atherosclerosis	COW, arteries
Arteriosclerosis	Small arteries, arterioles
Infarcts	Anywhere in the brain
• Micro	• Cortex, hippocampus
• Watershed	• Borders ACA, MCA, PCA
• Lacunes	• Thalamus, caudate, putamen
• Territorial	• Area of ACA, MCA, PCA
• Laminar necrosis	• Neocortex
Hemorrhage	Anywhere in the brain
• Micro	• Cortex, WM, basal ganglia
• Macro ICH	• Cerebrum, cerebellum
• SDH	• Subdural space
• SAH	• Subarachnoid space
• IVH	• Intraventricular rupture ICH
Amyloid angiopathy	Cortex, hippocampus and cerebellum, meninges and parenchyma
Aneurysms	COW
Vascular malformations	Cerebrum, cerebellum
Vasculitis/inflammation	Cerebrum, cerebellum, brainstem
CADASIL	Cerebrum
Binswanger's disease	Cerebral WM
Multi-infarct dementia	Cerebrum, basal ganglia, thalamus, WM, brainstem

(ACA: anterior cerebral artery; CADASIL: cerebral autosomal dominant arteriopathy with subcortical infarcts and leukoencephalopathy; COW: Circle of Willis; ICH: intracerebral hemorrhage; MCA: middle cerebral artery; PCA: posterior cerebral artery; WM: white matter.)

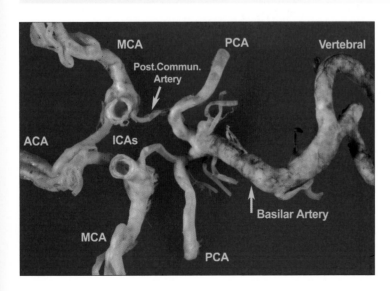

6.4 A complete Circle of Willis arterial tree shows yellow atherosclerotic plaques preferentially involving the posterior circulation (basilar artery; vertebral artery; posterior communicating artery). The major branches are labeled: ACA: anterior cerebral artery; MCA: middle cerebral artery; PCA: posterior cerebral artery; ICAs: internal carotid arteries. (Formalin fixed autopsy specimen.)

blood vessels from the middle cerebral artery (MCA). A subset of affected brains exhibit sparing of the COW with AS confined to end terminal arteries; this subtype is uncommon yet may pose the most risk of infarction to the patient. The hippocampus is particularly vulnerable to symptomatic infarctions due to terminal artery AS.

The basic pathologic lesion of all affected vessels is the intimal plaque (**6.5**). Aortic fatty streaks first develop during childhood. Subsequently, smooth muscle hyperplasia of the media occurs and foam cells (macrophages) infiltrate first the intima and then extend into the aortic media. These collective processes lead to thickening of the arterial wall with later fibrosis, intimal hyperplasia, and luminal narrowing. Such plaques may form in the aortic arch, break off, and act as emboli to the brain. Carotid artery plaques can narrow the lumen and, as in the arch, are recognized foci for thrombus formation. Severe, critical narrowing or unilateral carotid artery stenosis may be associated with cognitive impairment as the sole clinical symptom (Lehrner *et al.*, 2005). Intraplaque hemorrhages in the carotids or COW arteries can lead to abrupt luminal stenosis or occlusion, thereby precipitating an acute infarct (tissue death). Therapeutic administration of tissue plasminogen activator (TPA) can interrupt this sequence of events and is being widely employed during early stages of an incipient stroke (ischemic infarct). Unfortunately, TPA can itself cause severe or lethal intracerebral hemorrhage (Wang *et al.*, 2004).

6.5 An eccentric atherosclerotic fibrous plaque of a major Circle of Willis branch occludes the arterial lumen by about 30%, which is not sufficient to significantly impair blood flow. (H&E, ×1 objective.)

Arteriosclerosis

Arteriosclerosis refers to a constellation of pathologic changes that affect smaller arteries and arterioles. Historically, this spectrum of vascular pathology has been termed fibrohyalinosis, 'hypertensive vasculopathy', or 'fibrinoid necrosis' in persons with high blood pressure, or 'small vessel disease'. The overall effect is to constrict the vascular lumen and to cause a critical reduction of blood flow, the critical stenosis level, when luminal narrowing exceeds about 75% (**6.6**).

For the arterial blood supply to the heart, this threshold for producing ischemic symptoms from reduced coronary blood flow is referred to as critical coronary stenosis. Both the coronary and the cerebral arterial circulations have redundant collateral blood flow sources that mitigate the

---

Box 6.2 Cerebral small vessel disease

- CAA (cerebral amyloid angiopathy), spontaneous or with gene mutations in:
  - beta-amyloid precursor protein (Dutch type)
  - Cystatin C (island/Icelandic type)
  - Transthyretin
  - Gelsolin
- CAA in Alzheimer's disease (94.1%) and controls (33.3%)
- CADASIL (cerebral autosomal dominant arteriopathy with stroke and ischemic leukoencephalopathy), notch-3 gene mutations
- CARASIL (cerebral autosomal recessive arteriopathy with stroke and ischemic leukoencephalopathy)
- Hereditary cerebral microangiopathy (normal notch-3 gene)
- Ischemic leukoencephalopathy
- Degenerative cerebral microangiopathy
- Mitochondrial myopathy, encephalopathy, lactic-acidosis, and stroke-like episodes
- SUSAC'S syndrome (arterial occlusive syndrome with encephalopathy and retinal involvement)
- Retinocerebral vasculopathies
- Bleeding associated with Apo E ε2 allele

(Barker *et al.*, 1999; Jellinger, 2005; Ringelstein & Nabavi, 2005) effect of critical stenosis of a single main artery. The ultimate outcome result, that is, either no symptoms with no or reversible pathology, *versus* symptoms and irreversible pathology, is highly dependent on the time course over which critical arterial stenosis develops. This factor in turn affects the magnitude of the collateral circulatory capacity present at any given time. If the stenosis develops abruptly, for example by embolism or thrombosis, then the obstruction often produces infarction in the absence of compensatory mechanisms.

Infarcts

Death and later dissolution of brain tissue (encephalomalacia) occurs when blood flow drops below a critical perfusion threshold and autoregulation fails, or when sustained hypoxemia occurs (as in drowning or asphyxiation). A number of subtypes of cerebral infarcts are recognized. Many such lesions are clinically silent during life and are only appreciated on MRI scans or at autopsy.

Territorial macroinfarcts

Territorial macroinfarcts are larger than 1.5 cm in diameter and occur in major arterial territories supplied by a single artery or a segmental branch thereof. Thus, an infarct resulting from occlusion of the superficial branches of the MCA will cause damage (necrosis) to most of the dorsolateral cerebral cortex. Such infarcts may be: (1) acute, either ischemic (**6.7**) or hemorrhagic (**6.8**) and marked primarily by softening; (2) subacute with tissue necrosis (leukomalacia) (**6.9**); or (3) remote with cavitation, grossly visible atrophy of descending motor tracts (**6.10**), and major loss of brain volume (**6.11**). If the main MCA trunk is occluded, there may also be necrosis of the deeper branch territory in the basal ganglia and thalamus. The frontal and occipital poles supplied, respectively, by the anterior and posterior cerebral arteries, will be relatively spared assuming these other arteries are patent.

Bilateral medial occipital infarction is a common pattern seen when the posterior cerebral arteries are occluded by thrombosis or embolism (**6.12**). Occlusion of the arterial supply also produces isolated cerebellar infarcts (Milandre *et al.*, 1992). Such infarcts show loss of the folial architecture acutely and, after full evolution of the hypoxic ischemic insult, result in foci of microscopic internal granular cell and Purkinje neuron loss with secondary astrocytic gliosis (**6.13, 6.14**).

6.6 A: A complex, partly calcified atherosclerotic plaque almost completely occludes a cerebral artery. The tiny residual lumen contains a few red cells, but effective blood flow has ceased. (H&E, ×1 objective.) **B**: An organizing cerebral intra-arterial thrombus has recanalized. Multiple vascular lumens can be seen. This reparative process takes at least several weeks to occur. (H&E, ×10 objective.)

6.7 A coronal section through the prefrontal lobes of a recent middle cerebral artery, unilateral, ischemic infarct. The affected cortex (on the viewer's right) is discolored, slightly darker than the opposite hemisphere, and a faint geographic demarcation zone is apparent. The affected area has a green tinge because the patient was jaundiced. Such lesions are less firm when touched. (Formalin-fixed autopsy brain specimen.) (Courtesy of Dr Robert E Schmidt.)

6.8 A hemorrhagic infarct (on the viewer's left), at the same rostrocaudal coronal level, is shown for comparison to **6.7**. The infarcted zone is suffused with red blood that conforms mostly to the cortical gray matter ribbon with its richer vascular network compared to white matter. (Formalin-fixed autopsy brain specimen.) (Courtesy of Dr Robert E Schmidt.)

6.9 This coronal section shows a cavitating subacute infarct that involves the left caudate nucleus and internal capsule. Brain parenchyma has been liquefied and removed leaving visible voids in the tissue. The arrows point to bilateral probable and incidental white matter lacunes. (Formalin-fixed autopsy brain specimen.) (Courtesy of Dr Robert E Schmidt.)

6.10 This image array shows the long-term effect of a middle cerebral artery occlusion and resulting ischemic infarct. The axonal fibers of the long descending motor tracts have atrophied. As a result, the cerebral peduncles (mid-brain), the crossing fibers of the basis pontis, and the medullary pyramids of the brainstem (on viewer's left) derived from the infarcted hemisphere have atrophied. (Formalin fixed autopsy specimen.) (Courtesy of Dr Robert E Schmidt.)

6.11 A: The chronic effects of a large territorial left middle cerebral infarct are shown in sagittal (**A**) and coronal (**B**, yellow arrows) views. **A**: Much of the lateral convexity has disappeared leaving a ragged irregular surface. (Formalin fixed autopsy specimen.) **B**: Marked loss of the left hemisphere prefrontal lobe parenchyma. Remaining left hemisphere tissue is supplied by the intact anterior cerebral artery supply. Compare to the intact (noninfarcted) right hemisphere. The anterior cerebral arteries are free of atherosclerosis at this coronal level (black arrow). (Formalin fixed autopsy specimen.)

6.12 A bilateral infarct with multiple small foci of hemorrhage involves both medial occipital lobes. (Formalin fixed autopsy specimen.)

6.13 An evolving cerebellar ischemic infarct shows sharply defined geographic necrosis that spans gray and white matter of several adjacent folia. (H&E, ×1 objective.)

6.14 A more chronic cerebellar infarct exhibits advanced tissue dissolution compared to **6.13**. The occluded atherosclerotic artery that caused this lesion may be seen at lower right. (H&E, ×1 objective.)

6.15 A subacute microinfarct of the cerebral cortex spans the surfaces of two adjacent gyri. The underlying white matter shows pallor due to edema. (H&E, ×1 objective.)

Microinfarcts

Microinfarcts occur throughout the cerebral gray and white matter (**6.15**). One definition is infarcts that are 2 mm in diameter or less that are not appreciated grossly. Recently, microinfarction of cerebral cortex and hippocampus have been implicated as causes of cognitive impairment (Dinsdale *et al.*, 1971-2; Fein *et al.*, 2000; Miklossy, 2003; Kovari *et al.*, 2004). In contrast, McKee and the NACC Vascular Dementia Consortium report that cortical microinfarction is rare in 100 Massachusetts General Hospital AD patients (ADRC Core Leaders meeting June 23, 2004, unpublished data). The prevalence of dementia was correlated with small and large infarcts in the Nun study (Snowdon *et al.*, 1997). Participants with lacunar infarcts in the basal ganglia, thalamus, or deep WM were particularly at risk.

Watershed infarcts

These occur in brain overlap regions between the areas supplied by major branches of the COW: the anterior, middle, and posterior cerebral arteries. Recently, microinfarcts have been shown to occur preferentially in these same areas using a tissue histoblotting technique (Jendroska *et al.*, 1995). Using this sensitive technique it was possible to demonstrate watershed infarcts confined to watershed infarct zones.

Lacunar infarcts

Lacunes were defined by Fisher (1965, 1991) as small cerebral or cerebellar infarcts measuring 1.5 cm or less in greatest diameter. Lacunes that were greater than 1.0 cm in diameter were referred to as 'giant lacunes'. Small ones that occur in the preferred areas of the thalamus and basal ganglia must often be distinguished on MRI from dilated Virchow–Robins perivascular spaces (Longstreth *et al.*, 1998). Large-scale surveys of lacunar ischemic lesions have led to the recognition of several subtypes (*Tables 6.7, 6.8*)

Table 6.7 Types of cerebrovascular lacunae (small infarcts <1.5 cm diameter)

1a	result in clinical stroke syndromes
1b	silent lacunae
2	hemorrhagic lacune
3	dilatation of perivascular spaces

Subtypes – giant or expanding lacune (>1 cm diameter)

(Derouesne *et al.*, 1987; Challa & Moody, 1989; Derouesne & Poirier, 1999)

Table 6.8 Classical symptoms of pseudobulbar palsy (expected in lacunar state)

- Walking with small steps
- Episodes of laughing and crying
- Dysarthria
- Incontinence
- Imbalance

(Fisher, 1965 [Comte A. Des paralysies pseudobulbaires, Paris Thesis, 1900, No. 436])

(**6.16**, **6.17**). Such lacunes must be distinguished from dilated Virchow–Robins spaces by both pathologists (**6.18**) and neuroradiologists (Bokura *et al.*, 1998; Patankar *et al.*, 2005).

Laminar cortical necrosis

Laminar cortical necrosis (LCN) results from globally reduced blood flow, oxygenation, or both factors, of brain tissue. Cortical gray matter tissue is preferentially affected, resulting in necrosis of the middle cortical layers (Castillo *et al.*, 1996). Later, the necrotic areas are resorbed leaving a partly collapsed, vacuolated and gliotic region in the middle cortical laminae (**6.19**). The microscopic appearance is similar to other types of infarcts at similar stages of evolution, with polymorphonuclear leukocytes being common in acute stages, gitter macrophages and plump gemistocytic astrocytes in subacute stages, and cavitation and fibrillary astrocytosis in later stages (**6.20**). In extreme cases, the dead brain is totally resorbed leaving a slit-like hole that affects several adjacent millimeters of the cortical ribbon.

The cerebral cortex in advanced FTD features severe vacuolization (status spongiosus) that superficially resembles laminar necrosis. Both FTD and LCN cortices share astrocytic gliosis as a major lesion. The major microscopic features that define LCN in the acute and subacute phases are true necrosis and presence of lipid-rich macrophages ('gitter cells'). Neither lesion is part of the FTD spectrum. In addition, neuron loss in LCN is sharply demarcated and is confined to areas of necrosis. In contrast, neuron loss in FTD occurs throughout the cortical ribbon; particular laminae are affected at first in a patchy manner and later diffusely.

6.16 A: Small white lacunes (bottom arrow) are seen in the deep prefrontal white matter. The top arrow points to a cortical infarct. (Coronal section, formalin fixed autopsy specimen.) **B:** Caudate lacunes (yellow arrow) are one form of 'strategic' lacunes that have been reported to cause dementia. Black arrows denote atheroma lipid in anterior and middle cerebral arteries. (Formalin fixed autopsy specimen.) **C:** Pontine lacunes are common lesions of the elderly. This example shows typical uneven ('ragged') edges with fine residual fibrovascular tissue trabeculae traversing the lumen. A smaller satellite lacune is nearby to the left of the main lesion. (Formalin fixed autopsy specimen.) (**C** courtesy of Dr Robert E Schmidt.)

6.17 A: The fibrovascular stalk of a remote lacune consists of connective tissue surrounding several arterioles within the cavity of the infarct. H&E, ×10 objective. **B**: The wall of a subacute, weeks old lacune consists of foamy 'gitter cell' macrophages, neuropil, and enlarged gemistocytic astrocytes (gliosis). H&E, ×10 objective. **C**: A thalamic lacune that occasionally is associated with dementia. The demarcating necrotic focus is wedge-shaped with an irregular contour. H&E, ×1 objective. **D**: Contrast the histology of the cystic thalamic lacune in (**C**) with a more acute caudate nucleus lacune that has not yet cavitated. (H&E, ×1 objective.)

6.18 The ventral and posterior putamen, a subdivision of the basal ganglia, is a favorite location of dilated slit-like and oval to round Virchow–Robins (V-R) perivascular spaces (arrows) in the brain. Compared to lacunes of the same size, V-R spaces are usually smooth walled without internal trabeculae. (Formalin fixed autopsy specimen.)

6.19 A coronal section of prefrontal lobes shows two distinct types of lesions: a white matter lacune (yellow arrow) and a focus of cortical laminar necrosis (black arrow). The affected cortex shows slit-like concave necrosis due to tissue loss that follows the cortical ribbon curvature. (Formalin fixed autopsy specimen.)

6.20 A medium power view of the center of an evolving necrotic lacunar infarct is filled with foamy gitter cell macrophages. (H&E, ×20 objective.)

6.21 A recent hematoma excavates the left parietal–occipital lobe in a coronal section. The cerebral hemorrhage at autopsy is dark red, firm, and friable due to early organization and the hardening effects of formaldehyde chemical fixation. The other hemisphere has a nonhemorrhagic infarct. Autopsy specimen of an Alzheimer brain which also had severe cerebral amyloid angiopathy. (Formalin fixed autopsy specimen.)

6.22 A: A subacute partly organized cerebellar hemisphere hemorrhage is seen ventral to the occipital lobe in this lateral view of the cerebrum. (Formalin fixed autopsy specimen.) **B**: The same cerebellar hemisphere hemorrhage shown in (**A**) as it appears on the ventral surface of the brain. The medulla has been transected during brain removal. SC: spinal cord. The arrow points to the basilar artery. (Formalin fixed autopsy specimen.)

Hemorrhage

Hemorrhage caused by ruptured blood vessels (usually arteries) or aneurysms (arterial wall dilatations) may be acute (hours to days), subacute (1–3 weeks) or chronic (greater than 3 weeks to months or years old) (Fisher, 1971). Cerebral (**6.21**), cerebellar (**6.22**) and brainstem hemorrhages may be large (several millimeters to centimeters in diameter) or microscopically small, i.e. microhemorrhages (**6.23**, **6.24**). Risk factors for cerebral hemorrhage are presented in *Table 6.9*.

Macrohemorrhages

Macrohemorrhages are grossly visible areas of bleeding that are subdural, subarachnoid, parenchymal, or intra-ventricular. Hemorrhage size and location are critically dependent on the specific etiology that led to bleeding.

Intracerebral and cerebellar hemorrhage (ICH). Risk and etiologic factors that determine size and location of central nervous system (CNS) parenchymal bleeding include the following examples: fat embolism centered on the cortical

Table 6.9 Cerebral hemorrhage risk factors
• Cerebral amyloid angiopathy
• Apolipoprotein E, ε4 allele
• Hypertension
• Trauma
• Vasculitis (inflammatory vascular disease)
• Microaneurysms
• Fibrinoid necrosis of the vessel wall
(Vonsattel *et al.*, 1991)

gray–white matter junction seen as petechiae several millimeters in diameter; hypertension (basal ganglia, thalamus, cerebellum), cerebellar tonsillar hemorrhage in cerebral edema with tonsillar herniation, and cerebral brainstem compression with secondary hemorrhages in the mid-brain and pons (termed Duret hemorrhages).

6.23 An acute subdural hemorrhage shows five foci of clotted blood adhering to the undersurface of the dura which has been removed in pieces. (Formalin fixed autopsy specimen.)

6.24 Cross-section of a chronic (organized) subdural hemorrhage which has formed a fibrous pseudomembrane. Myxofibrous translucent tissue separates the dura and the subdural pseudomembrane. (Formalin fixed autopsy specimen.)

Intraventricular hemorrhage (IVC). Most ventricular hemorrhages are secondary extensions from parenchymal hemorrhages. Emergency surgery is frequently required to decompress the brain by evacuating the original parenchymal or ventricular hematomas. Microscopic examination of the clot can reveal the age of the hemorrhage. Acute hemorrhages consist primarily of intact red blood cells with small amounts of fibrin. Subacute (weeks old) and chronic hemorrhages (months) post-evacuation show varying degrees of lysis and organization marked by the presence of fibroblastic infiltration and gitter cell macrophages.

Subdural hemorrhage (SDH). Traumatic SDHs in the cognitively intact elderly are primarily due to falling. Demented patients with AD and Lewy disorders often have repeated falling episodes, and thus are at even greater risk for developing SDH. It is likely that a portion of falls in 'healthy aging' occur in people with preclinical AD or incipient dementia that is undetected before the fall or head trauma occurs. Acute SDH appear as fresh blood clots or hematomas (**6.23**). Remote SDH develop a thick pseudomembrane that organizes and becomes fused to the dura (**6.24**).

Subarachnoid hemorrhage (SAH). Trauma, often due to falls, is the most common cause of SAH in the elderly. In contrast, SAH in younger individuals is most often secondary to a ruptured Berry aneurysm. Similar to SDH, acute hemorrhages contain intact red blood cells (RBCs), whereas organized hematomas are the rule later on. SAH may be confined to the leptomeninges or may rupture into the cerebral or cerebellar parenchyma and the ventricles.

Microhemorrhages

Microhemorrhages are perivascular extravasation of RBCs that may be acute (**6.25**) or chronic (**6.26**). Acute perivascular hemorrhages may be confined to the bounds of the Virchow–Robins spaces or may extend into the brain parenchyma. It is often difficult to distinguish between a simple hemorrhage and a hemorrhagic infarct. Recent neuroimaging studies have focused both MRI (T2* and similar sequences) (Imaizumi *et al.*, 2005) and positron emission tomography (PET) (Mielke & Heiss, 1998) techniques to visualize minute foci of cerebral bleeding and hypometabolism due to infarction. MRI scan modalities have documented an association of microhemorrhagic foci with both hypertension (Fisher, 1971) and amyloid angiopathy (Lee & Stemmerman, 1978; van den Boom *et al.*, 2005).

6.25 An acute cerebral cortical hemorrhage is seen in a thioflavine S stained Alzheimer brain specimen. The ball-shaped hemorrhage seen at the left of the figure consists of intact red cells that have suffused into the surrounding brain parenchyma. Circular, brightly fluorescent profiles are amyloid-laden leptomeningeal and parenchymal arteries. Less intensely staining senile plaques are also apparent. (Fluorescence microscopy, thioflavine S stain, ×10 objective.)

6.26 A deep white matter artery is surrounded by inflammatory cells and macrophages containing golden brown hemoglobin pigment. The latter feature identifies this as the site of a previous, remote microhemorrhage. (H&E, ×10 objective.)

Microhemorrhages, if chronic, may appear at autopsy as relatively normal gray or white matter small arteries or arterioles that are surrounded by a few pigmented macrophages. Use of iron stains (Perl's method or ferritin immunostaining, for example) may reveal iron pigment within macrophage cytoplasm, indicating RBCs have lysed leaving iron-rich heme pigment.

Cerebral amyloid angiopathy (CAA)

Deposition of beta-amyloid protein is a crucial lesion that can contribute to cognitive impairment and dementia. CAA may occur as an isolated lesion during normal aging, or can co-occur with AD and other dementias (Lippa et al., 1993; Olichney et al., 2000). CAA deposition in leptomeningeal vessels has also been implicated in causing WM dysfunction (Gray et al., 1985; Roher et al., 2003). CAA is usually not a macroscopically visible lesion. Microscopically, hematoxylin and eosin (H&E) routine sections show thickened arterial or arteriolar walls that may be focally acellular and may have a double lumen (**6.27**). The latter lesion was first described by Romanul and Abramowicz (Romanul & Abramowicz, 1964) in leptomeningeal arteries surrounding old infarcts. Microscopic examination of CAA shows a-beta protein deposition in the vascular wall (**6.28**).

The following three disorders are uncommon causes of progressive dementia. The relevant pathology is briefly mentioned here for the sake of completeness.

Aneurysms

Aneurysms are abnormally dilated segments of arteries that occur when the arterial wall is weakened congenitally (Berry aneurysm) or by a pathologic process (medial necrosis, AS, infection). Charcot–Bouchard aneurysms result from arteriosclerotic processes (Challa et al., 1992). Microaneurysms, also referred to as miliary aneurysms, are commonly seen in lacunes (Fisher, 1969), in brains from patients with diabetes mellitus (DeJong, 1977), and in hypertensive brains (Anim & Kofi, 1984) (**6.29**).

Vascular malformations

Congenital vascular lesions may be composed of arteries, veins, and microvascular components occurring alone or in combination (Zabramski et al., 2005). Rarely do these lesions contribute materially to dementia.

6.27 Multiple leptomeningeal arteries in the depths of a cerebral sulcus exhibit a double wall with a clear space in between. Such 'double barrel lumen' (DBL) blood vessels were first described by Romanul and Abramowicz (1964). DBL vessels are usually the site of amyloid angiopathy in brains from elderly controls and Alzheimer patients. (H&E, ×10 objective.)

6.28 Beta-amyloid deposition (brown vascular profiles) is shown involving the walls of cerebellar meningeal arteries. Most of the field is occupied by the molecular layer neuropil. (A-beta antibody-diaminobenzidine [DAB, brown] immunohistochemical stain, ×10 objective.)

6.29 A: A typical diabetic or hypertensive (miliary) microaneurysm in the leptomeninges has the same morphology as ones occurring in the subcortex. The blood vessel wall is focally dilated and the lumen contains material that could represent organized fibrin thrombus with atherosclerotic plaque. Note slit-like cholesterol clefts are present. (H&E, ×1 objective.) **B**: A similar microaneurysmal arterial lesion reveals argyrophilic material that is more layered compared to the lesion shown in (**A**). (Modified Bielschowsky silver method, ×1 objective.)

Vasculitis and inflammation

Patients with dementia are subject to systemic infectious and inflammatory disorders that may involve the brain. Such disorders are listed in *Table 6.6*. The following discussions briefly review only the vascular contributions of these disorders to dementia, recognizing that the probability of causation ranges from minimal and nonspecific to severe and pathognomonic.

Systemic lupus erythematosus (SLE). Neuropsychiatric SLE with dementia is a well recognized disorder (Hanly, 2005). Lacunar infarcts may result from lupus-induced vascular thromboembolism associated with circulating anticoagulants (Hanly *et al.*, 1992). Cerebral microangiopathy, vasculitis, heart emboli that may affect the brain, and thrombotic thrombocytopenic purpura (TTP) are recognized complications of SLE that lead to cerebral infarction and affect cognition and brain function, including seizure induction. MRI findings in SLE include macroinfarction, microinfarction, and diffuse signal intensity areas of dysfunctional cortex (Aisen *et al.*, 1985).

Progressive multifocal leukoencephalopathy (PML). The human JC virus causes bizarre astrocytic glial inclusions accompanied by WM demyelination and axon loss in the severe form. Lesions tend to be vasocentric. Patients usually are debilitated from chronic or infectious disorders such as aquired immunodeficiency syndrome/human immunodeficiency virus (AIDS/HIV) (Cinque *et al.*, 2003).

AIDS-HIV. People with chronic HIV infection may become demented due to either a primary encephalopathy or to the combined effects of secondary infectious diseases involving the CNS. Thirty percent of cortical neurons and hippocampal neurons may be lost (Korbo & West, 2000), and this factor can contribute to cognitive dysfunction and cerebral atrophy seen on brain scans.

Viral infections. Many types of viruses cause acute or subacute encephalitis, with transient confusion or cognitive impairment. With the exception of HIV, however, such virus-associated cognitive impairments rarely lead to chronic dementia.

Bacterial infections. Tertiary neural syphilis, a spirochetal disease caused by *Treponema pallidum*, which is now rarely encountered, commonly causes a progressive dementing disorder during the terminal phase.

Fungal infections. Certain fungi, particularly *Aspergillus*, *Mucor*, and *Candida*, may invade and damage cerebral blood vessels. Released procoagulants may cause secondary thrombotic infarction or intracerebral hemorrhages. Subacute mental confusion and occasionally dementia may ensue.

Meningitis

Elderly institutionalized patients are a recognized high-risk group for developing bacterial (beta-streptococcal) meningitis. The authors have encountered three recent severely demented AD patients who developed a terminal acute beta-streptococcal (culture-confirmed) acute meningitis that was unrecognized clinically prior to death. Acute meningeal and superficial neutrophilic invasive lesions were superimposed on the chronic plaque and tangle lesions of AD. Polymorphonuclear leucocytes prominently surrounded meningeal arteries. Tubercular infections with *Mycobacterium tuberculosis* cause a basal meningitis that causes an obliterative endovasculitis. Occluded basilar arteries lead to secondary infarction.

Histiocytosis-X (synonyms: Hand–Schuller–Christian disease, Abt–Letterer–Siwe disease, eosinophilic granulomas of bone)

In this disease, a chronic inflammatory, vasocentric cellular infiltrate often involves the hypothalamus and basal forebrain. The disorder usually occurs in children and is only an occasional cause of adult dementia.

Amebic/parasitic infections

A wide variety of amebic and parasitic infections can cause a chronic cerebritis and vasculitis. These include cysticercosis, amebiasis, and borreliosis which, when they become chronic, can impair cognition.

CADASIL

Cerebral autosomal dominant arteriopathy with subcortical infarcts and leukoencephalopathy (CADASIL) is a dementing neurologic disorder that features recurring cerebral infarcts and hemorrhages associated with a distinctive vasculopathy in relatively young patients (Kalaria et al., 2004; Lesnik et al., 2004). Many of the cases are hereditary and are associated with a mutation in the Notch 3 gene located on chromosome 19. The WM may show macroscopic areas of necrosis similar to Binswanger's disease (**6.30**). However, most CADASIL patients are normotensive. The diagnostic finding in cerebral blood vessels are mural thickening and deposition in the medial layer of electron dense granular material that may be seen by either H&E (**6.31A**) or periodic acid-Schiff (PAS) stains (**6.31B**).

6.30 A hemicoronal section of parietal lobe from a CADASIL patient reveals multiple deep white matter infarcts (WMI) (arrows). WMI appear as rough textured, sunken areas in the formalin fixed white matter. (Formalin fixed autopsy specimen.) (Courtesy of Dr Robert E Schmidt.)

6.31 A: CADASIL artery with diagnostic eosinophilic granular material in the media. (H&E, ×10 objective.) **B**: Another CADASIL case blood vessel in which the diagnostic medial granular material is visualized using the periodic acid-Schiff (PAS) stain. (PAS-hematoxlin, ×10 objective.)

Binswanger's disease

This disorder was originally described as an ischemic disorder with widespread grossly visible WM infarcts (Binswanger, 1894; Fisher, 1989). The pathologic lesion spectrum is expressed in the original name: subacute arteriosclerotic subcortical dementia. Current recognition as a coherent clinicopathologic entity remains clouded by lack of validated reliable neuropathologic criteria, compounded by a confusion caused by MRI lesions consisting of abnormal signal intensity that occur commonly in the nondemented elderly and in Alzheimer patients (Longstreth *et al.*, 1996; Tomimoto *et al.*, 1999; van Dijk *et al.*, 2002). Such lesions often reveal only edema when examined by a pathologist, and hence do not correspond to the lesions that Binswanger originally described. In the authors' experience, multiple grossly visible WM infarcts that completely spare the cortex are rare findings in dementia brains. One example from a sibling pair with early-onset dementia, a non-CADASIL hereditary leukoencephalopathy, and multifocal CAA, is shown in **6.32, 6.33**.

Multi-infarct dementia (MID)

Some demented people experience a series of cerebral infarcts in gray and white matter. MID was first studied in a meaningful way as a possible cause of dementia by Tomlinson *et al.* (1968; 1970). These investigators showed that most cases of dementia were associated with AD plaques and tangles rather than vascular disease (strokes). Further, they concluded that relatively large amounts of brain tissue (50–100 ml) had to be destroyed in order to cause dementia. Subsequent experience with intensively studied stroke patients, including the use of neuroimaging to describe the full extent of infarcts, has shown that many large territorial infarcts are usually accompanied by mild cognitive changes rather than overt dementia (Mackowiak-Cordoliani *et al.*, 2005; Rasquin *et al.*, 2005). Dementia prevalence and incidence were variable depending on the diagnostic criteria used. Prevalence was 11.3% (NINDS–AIREN) to 20.1% (ICD-10-NA); incidence was 2.6% (ADDTC) to 5.2% (ICD-10-NA) (see *Table 6.1*). Imaging has also confirmed autopsy series showing that many smaller infarcts may be clinically silent (Shinkawa *et al.*, 1995).

A recently studied case at the authors' center was particularly informative on the issue of infarction and dementia. An 89-year-old woman was followed over 6 years until death. Postmortem CDR was 0.5, indicating very mild dementia. No AD pathology was found at autopsy despite use of a-beta and tau immunostaining. Rather, the 1050 g brain contained 19 separate infarcts ranging in size from 0.2–2.5 cm in diameter.

Current clinical emphasis is trending towards identifying small vessel disease and resulting cortical microinfarcts and WM MRI lesions as the underlying cause of ischemic vascular cognitive impairment (Jellinger, 2002b; de Mendonca *et al.*, 2005). Many studies in this field still suffer from a paucity of autopsy confirmed series. For example, many WM lesion studies which lack autopsy data state the lesions were due to 'small vessel disease'. Yet, direct characterization of co-registered anatomic brain slices and MRI images have generally focused on edema as the cause of periventricular MRI 'caps'. Pathologists are often surprised that areas of deep WM with dramatic MRI hyperintensities grossly appear normal in freshly sectioned or fixed brains. Microscopy rarely reveals frank infarcts. Edema resulting in myelin pallor, myelin loss, rare axonal damage, and occasional loss of oligodendrocytes and macrophage accumulation and vascular wall thickening and hyalinization may be seen. This set of findings often falls short of the pathologic lesion profile that Brun and Englund (1986) termed 'incomplete infarction'.

In summary, it is quite clear that vascular dementia must be considered in light of aging-related vascular anatomy, hypertensive effects on cerebral blood vessels, and multiple complications of arteriosclerosis and AS as they interplay with the clinical expression of AD and related dementing disorders. It is probable, therefore, that vascular factors play some contributing role in all of the dementing syndromes, and that pure VaD is a truly rare clinicopathologic entity.

6.32 Three mid-level coronal sections through the brain of one of two siblings who in their 40s developed a severe familial leukoencephalopathy of the Binswanger or 'vanishing white matter' phenotype. Affected gelatinous white matter (WM) (arrows) appears tan and translucent due to marked loss of both axons and myelin. The degeneration pattern of WM is geographic and closely tracks contours of the gray–white matter junction. (Formalin fixed autopsy specimen.)

6.33 A: Sections of gray–white matter junction from the same brain specimen illustrated in **6.32** have been stained to demonstrate severe loss of deep white matter (WM) myelin with relative preservation of the subcortical U-fibers (arrows define the U-fibers and damaged WM to the right). GM: gray matter cortex. (Luxol fast blue-Periodic acid-Schiff [LFB-PAS] [Kluver-Barrera] stain, ×10 objective.) **B**: Sections of gray–white matter junction from the same case illustrated in **6.32** have been stained to demonstrate the severe loss of deep WM axons with relative preservation of the subcortical U-fibers (middle of figure). The rarified white matter is positioned on the left. An ependymal surface is to the right of the figure. (Gallyas silver method, ×10 objective.)

References

Aisen AM, Gabrielsen TO, McCune WJ (1985). MR imaging of systemic lupus erythematosus involving the brain. *Am. J. Roentgenol.* **144**:1027–1031.

American Psychiatric Association (1994). *Diagnostic and Statistical Manual of Mental Disorders, Fourth Edition (DSM-IV)*. American Psychiatric Association, Washington, DC, pp. 143–147.

Anim JT, Kofi AD (1984). Hypertension, cerebral vascular changes and stroke in Ghana. 1. Microaneurysm formation and stroke. *J. Pathol.* **143**:177–182.

Barker RA, Anderson JR, Meyer P, *et al.* (1999). Microangiopathy of the brain and retina with hearing loss in a 50-year-old woman: extending the spectrum of Susac's syndrome. *J. Neurol. Neurosurg. Psych.* **66**:641–643.

Berg L, McKeel DW Jr, Miller JP, *et al.* (1998). Clinicopathologic studies in cognitively healthy aging and Alzheimer disease: relation of histologic markers to dementia severity, age, sex, and apolipoprotein E genotype. *Arch. Neurol.* **55**:326–335.

Bernick C, Kuller L, Dulberg C, *et al.* (2001). Silent MRI infarcts and the risk of future stroke: the cardiovascular health study. *Neurology* **57**:1222–1229.

Binswanger O (1894). Die abgrenzung der algemeinen progressiven paralyse (Referat, erstattet auf der Jahresversammlung des Vereins Deutscher Irrenärzte zu Dresden am 20 Sept. 1894). *Berl. Klin. Wochschr.* **31**:1103–1105;1137–1139;1180–1186.

Bokura H. Kobayashi S. Yamaguchi S (1998). Distinguishing silent lacunar infarction from enlarged Virchow–Robin spaces: a magnetic resonance imaging and pathological study. [See comment.] *J. Neurol.* **245**(2):116–122.

Brun A, Englund E (1986). A white matter disorder in dementia of the Alzheimer type: a pathoanatomical study. *Ann. Neurol.* **19**:253–262.

Brust JCM (1983). Vascular dementia: still overdiagnosed. *Stroke* **140**:298–300.

Castillo M, Scatliff JH, Kwock L, *et al.* (1996). Postmortem MR imaging of lobar cerebral infarction with pathologic and in vivo correlation. *Radiographics* **16**:241–250.

Challa VR, Moody DM (1989). The value of magnetic resonance imaging in the detection of type II hemorrhagic lacunes. *Stroke* **20**(6):822–825.

Challa VR, Moody DM, Bell MA (1992). The Charcot–Bouchard aneurysm controversy: impact of a new histologic technique.[See comment.] *J. Neuropathol. Exp. Neurol.* **51**:264–271.

Chui HC, Mack W, Jackson JE, *et al.* (2000). Clinical criteria for the diagnosis of vascular dementia: a multicenter study of comparability and interrater reliability.[see comment]. *Arch. Neurol.* **57**:191–196.

Chui HC, Victoroff JI, Margolin D, *et al.* (1992). Criteria for the diagnosis of ischemic vascular dementia proposed by the State of California Alzheimer's Disease Diagnostic and Treatment Centers. *Neurology* **42**:473–480.

Cinque P, Bossolasco S, Brambilla AM, *et al.* (2003). The effect of highly active antiretroviral therapy-induced immune reconstitution on development and outcome of progressive multifocal leukoencephalopathy: study of 43 cases with review of the literature. [Review] *J. Neurovirol.* **9**(Suppl 1):73–80.

DeJong RN (1977). CNS manifestations of diabetes mellitus. *Postgrad. Med.* **61**:101–107.

de la Torre JC (2004). Alzheimer's disease is a vasocognopathy: a new term to describe its nature. (Review) (113 refs) *Neurol. Res.* **26**:517–524.

del Ser T, Bermejo F, Portera A, *et al.* (1990). Vascular dementia: a clinicopathological study. *J. Neurol. Sci.* **96**:1–17.

de Mendonca A, Ribeiro F, Guerreiro M, *et al.* (2005). Clinical significance of subcortical vascular disease in patients with mild cognitive impairment. *Eur. J. Neurol.* **12**(2):125–130.

Derouesne C, Gray F, Escourolle R, *et al.* (1987). 'Expanding cerebral lacunae' in a hypertensive patient with normal pressure hydrocephalus. *Neuropathol. Appl. Neurobiol.* **13**:309–320.

Derouesne C, Poirier J (1999). Cerebral lacunae: still a matter of debate. *Revue Neurologique* **155**(10):823–831.

Desmond DW (2004). The neuropsychology of vascular cognitive impairment: is there a specific cognitive deficit? *J. Neurol Sci.* **226**:3–7.

Dinsdale HB, Robertson DM, Chiang TY, *et al.* (1971–2). Hypertensive cerebral microinfarction and cerebrovascular reactivity. *Eur. Neurol.* **6**:29–33.

Fein G, Di Sclafani V, Tanabe J, *et al.* (2000). Hippocampal and cortical atrophy predict dementia in subcortical ischemic vascular disease. *Neurology* 55:1626–1635.

Fischer P, Jellinger K, Cardenas V, *et al.* (1991). Prospective neuropathological validation of Hachinski's Ischaemic Score in dementias. *J. Neurol. Neurosurg. Psych.* **54**:580–583.

Fisher CM (1965). Lacunes: small, deep cerebral infarcts. *Neurology* **15**:774–784.

Fisher CM (1969). The arterial lesions underlying lacunes. *Acta Neuropathol.* (Berl) **12**:1–15.

Fisher CM (1971). Pathological observations in hypertensive cerebral hemorrhage. *J. Neuropathol. Exp. Neurol.* **39**:536–550.

Fisher CM (1989). Binswanger's encephalopathy: a review. *J. Neurol.* **236**:65–79.

Fisher CM (1991). Lacunar infarcts: a review. *Cerebrovasc. Dis.* **1**:311–320.

Fratiglioni L, Launer LJ, Andersen K, *et al.* (2000). Neurologic Diseases in the Elderly Research Group. Incidence of dementia and major subtypes in Europe: a collaborative study of population-based cohorts. *Neurology* **54**(11, Suppl 5):S10–S15.

Garrett, KD, Browndyke JN, Whelihan, W, *et al.* (2004). The neuropsychological profile of vascular cognitive impairment-no dementia: comparisons to patients at risk for cerebrovascular disease and vascular dementia. *Arch. Clin. Neuropsychol.* **19**: 745–757.

Graham, NL, Emery T, Hodges JR (2004). Distinctive cognitive profiles in Alzheimer's disease and subcortical vascular dementia. *J. Neurol. Neurosurg. Psych.* **75**: 61–71.

Gray F, Dubas F, Roullet E, *et al.* (1985). Leukoencephalopathy in diffuse haemorrhagic cerebral amyloid angiopathy. *Ann. Neurol.* **18**:54–59.

Hachinski VC, Iliff LD, Zilhka E, *et al.* (1975). Cerebral blood flow in dementia. *Arch. Neurol.* **32**:632–637.

Hanly JG (2005). Neuropsychiatric lupus. (Review) (146 refs) *Rheum. Dis. Clin. N. Am.* **31**:273–298.

Hanly JG, Walsh NM, Sangalang V (1992). Brain pathology in systemic lupus erythematosus. *J. Rheumatol.* **19**:732–741.

Heyman A, Filenbaum GG, Welsh-Bohmer KA, *et al.* (1998). Cerebral infarcts in patients with autopsy-proven Alzheimer's disease: CERAD, part XVIII. *Neurology* **51**:159–162.

Hulette C, Nochlin D, McKeel DW Jr, *et al.* (1997). Clinical-neuropathologic findings in multi-infarct dementia: a report of six autopsied cases. *Neurology* **48**:668–672.

Ikeda M, Fukuhara R, Shigenobu K, *et al.* (2004). Dementia associated mental and behavioural disturbances in elderly people in the community: findings from the first Nakayama study. *J. Neurol. Neurosurg. Psych.* **75**:146–148.

Imaizumi T, Honma T, Horita Y, *et al.* (2005). Dot-like hemosiderin spots are associated with past hemorrhagic strokes in patients with lacunar infarcts. *J. Neuroimaging* **15**:157–163.

Jellinger KA (2002a). Alzheimer disease and cerebrovascular pathology: an update. (Review) (121 refs) *J. Neurol. Transmission* **109**:813–836.

Jellinger KA (2002b). The pathology of ischemic-vascular dementia: an update. (Review) (41 refs) *J. Neurol. Sci.* **203–204**:153–157.

Jellinger KA, Attems J (2005). Prevalence and pathogenic role of cerebrovascular lesions in Alzheimer disease. *J. Neurol. Sci.* **229–230**:37–41.

Jellinger KA, Mitter-Ferstl E (2003). The impact of cerebrovascular lesions in Alzheimer disease. A comparative autopsy study. *J. Neurol.* **250**:1050–1055.

Jendroska K, Poewe W, Daniel SE, *et al.* (1995). Ischemic stress induces deposition of amyloid beta immunoreactivity in human brain. *Acta Neuropath.* **90**:461–466.

Kalaria RN, Viitanen M, Kalimo H, *et al.* (2004). CADASIL Group of Vas-Cog. The pathogenesis of CADASIL: an update. (Review) (35 refs) *J. Neurol. Sci.* **226**:35–39.

Knopman DS, DeKosky ST, Cummings JL, *et al.* (2001). Practice parameter: diagnosis of dementia (an evidence-based review). Report of the Quality Standards Subcommittee of the American Academy of Neurology. (See comments) *Neurology* **56**:1143–1153.

Kovari E, Gold G, Herrmann FR, *et al.* (2004). Cortical microinfarcts and demyelination significantly affect cognition in brain aging. *Stroke* **35**:410–414.

Korbo L, West M (2000). No loss of hippocampal neurons in AIDS patients. *Acta Neuropathol.* **99**:529–533.

Korczyn AD (2005). The underdiagnosis of the vascular contribution to dementia. *J. Neurol. Sci.* **229–230**:3–6.

Lee SS, Stemmerman GN (1978). Congophilic angiopathy and cerebral hemorrhage. *Arch. Pathol. Lab. Med.* **102**:317–321.

Lehrner J, Willfort A, Mlekusch I, *et al.* (2005). Neuropsychological outcome 6 months after unilateral carotid stenting. *J. Clin. Exp. Neuropsychol.* **27**:859–866.

Lesnik, Oberstein SA, Haan J (2004). Cerebral autosomal dominant arteriopathy with subcortical infarcts and leukoencephalopathy (CADASIL). (Review) (87 refs) *Panminerva Medica* **46**:265–276.

Lindeboom J, Weinstein H (2004). Neuropsychology of cognitive ageing, minimal cognitive impairment, Alzheimer's disease, and vascular cognitive impairment. (Review) (12 refs) *Eur. J. Pharmacol.* **490**:83–86.

Lippa CF, Hamos JE, Smith TW, *et al.* (1993). Vascular amyloid deposition in Alzheimer's disease. Neither necessary nor sufficient for the local formation of plaques or tangles. *Arch. Neurol.* **50**:1088–1092.

Longstreth WT Jr, Bernick C, Manolio TA, *et al.* (1998). Lacunar infarcts defined by magnetic resonance imaging of 3660 elderly people. The Cardiovascular Health Study. *Arch. Neurol.* **55**:1217–1225.

Longstreth WT Jr, Manolio TA, Arnold A, *et al.* (1996). Clinical correlates of white matter findings on cranial magnetic resonance imaging of 3301 elderly people. The Cardiovascular Health Study. *Stroke* **27**:1274–1282.

Lopez OL, Kuller LH, Becker JT, *et al.* (2005). Classification of vascular dementia in the Cardiovascular Health Study Cognition Study. *Neurology* **64**:1539–1547.

Loring DW, Meador KJ, Mahurin RK, *et al.* (1986). Neuropsychological performance in dementia of the Alzheimer type and multi-infarct dementia. *Arch. Clin. Neuropsychol.* **1**:335–340.

Mackowiak-Cordoliani MA, Bombois S, Memin A, *et al.* (2005). Poststroke dementia in the elderly. *Drugs & Aging* **22**:483–493.

McPherson SE, Cummings JL (1996). Neuropsychological aspects of vascular dementia. *Brain & Cognition* **31**:269–282.

Mielke R, Heiss WD (1998). Positron emission tomography for diagnosis of Alzheimers-disease and vascular dementia. *J. Neural Transmission* Supplementum **53**:237–250.

Miklossy J (2003). Cerebral hypoperfusion induces cortical watershed microinfarcts which may further aggravate cognitive decline in Alzheimer's disease. (Review) (63 refs) *Neurol. Res.* **25**:605–610.

Milandre L, Brosset C, Gouirand R, *et al.* (1992). Pure cerebellar infarction. Thirty cases. *Presse Med.* **21**:1562–1565.

Moossy J (1993). Pathology of cerebral atherosclerosis. Influence of age, race, and gender. *Stroke* **24**(Suppl. 1):122–123.

Moroney JT, Bagiella E, Desmond DW, *et al.* (1997a). Meta-analysis of the Hachinski Ischemic Score in pathologically verified dementias. *Neurology* **49**:1096–1105.

Moroney JT, Bagiella E, Hachinski VC, *et al.* (1997b). Misclassification of dementia subtype using the Hachinski Ischemic Score: results of a meta-analysis of patients with pathologically verified dementias. *Ann. N.Y. Acad. Sci.* **826**:490–492.

Nolan KA, Lino MM, Seligmann AW, *et al.* (1998). Absence of vascular dementia in an autopsy series from a dementia clinic. *J. Am. Geriatr. Soc.* **46**:597–604.

Olichney JM, Hansen LA, Lee JH, *et al.* (2000). Relationship between severe amyloid angiopathy, apolipoprotein E genotype, and vascular lesions in Alzheimer's disease. (Review) (31 refs) *Ann. N.Y. Acad. Sci.* **903**:138–143.

Patankar TF, Mitra D, Varma A, *et al.* (2005). Dilatation of the Virchow–Robin space is a sensitive indicator of cerebral microvascular disease: a study in elderly patients with dementia. *Am. J. Neuroradiol.* **26**:1512–1520.

Rasquin SM, Lodder J, Verhey FR (2005). The effect of different diagnostic criteria on the prevalence and incidence of post-stroke dementia. *Neuroepidemiology* **24**:189–195.

Ringelstein EB, Nabavi DG (2005). Cerebral small vessel diseases: cerebral microangiopathies. (Review) (86 refs) *Curr. Opin. Neurol.* **18**:179–188.

Rockwood K, Pargad I, Hacinski V, *et al.* (1994). Consortium of Canadian Centres for Clinical Cognitive Research consensus statement. *Can. J. Neurol. Sci.* **21**:358–364.

Roher AE, Kuo YM, Esh C, *et al.* (2003). Cortical and leptomeningeal cerebrovascular amyloid and white matter pathology in Alzheimer's disease. *Mol. Med.* **9**:112–122.

Roman GC (2004). Vascular dementia. Advances in nosology, diagnosis, treatment and prevention. (Review) (92 refs) *Panminerva Medica* **46**:207–215.

Roman GC, Tatemichi TK, Erkinjuntti T, *et al.* (1993). Vascular dementia: diagnostic criteria for research studies: report of the NINDS-AIREN International Workshop. *Neurology* **43**:250–260.

Romanul FC, Abramowicz A (1964). Changes in brain and pial vessels in arterial border zones; a study of 13 cases. *Arch. Neurol.* **11**:40–65.

Rosen WG, Terry RD, Fuld PA, *et al.* (1980). Pathological verification of ischemic score in differentiation of dementias. *Ann. Neurol.* **7**:486–488.

Sachdev PS, Brodaty H, Valenzuela MJ, *et al.* (2004). The neuropsychological profile of vascular cognitive impairment in stroke and TIA patients. *Neurology* **62**(6):912–919.

Shinkawa A, Ueda K, Kiyohara Y, *et al.* (1995). Silent cerebral infarction in a community-based autopsy series in Japan. The Hisayama Study. *Stroke* **26**:380–385.

Snowdon DA, Greiner LH, Mortimer JA, *et al.* (1997). Brain infarction and the clinical expression of Alzheimer disease. *JAMA* **277**:813–817.

Tomimoto H, Akiguchi I, Akiyama H, *et al.* (1999). Vascular changes in white matter lesions of Alzheimer's disease. *Acta Neuropathol.* **97**:629–634.

Tomlinson BE, Blessed G, Roth M (1968). Observations on the brains of nondemented old people. *J. Neurol. Sci.* **7**:331–356.

Tomlinson BE, Blessed G, Roth M (1970). Observations on the brains of demented old people. *J. Neurol. Sci.* **11**:205–242.

van den Boom R, Bornebroek M, Behloul F, *et al.* (2005). Microbleeds in hereditary cerebral hemorrhage with amyloidosis-Dutch type. *Neurology* **64**:1288–1289.

van Dijk EJ, Prins ND, Vermeer SE, *et al.* (2002). Frequency of white matter lesions and silent lacunar infarcts. (Review) (61 refs) *J. Neural Transmission Supplementum* **62**:25–39.

Verhey F, Lodder J, Rozendaal N, *et al.* (1996). Comparison of seven sets of criteria used for the diagnosis of vascular dementia. *Neuroepidemiology* **15**:16–72.

Vonsattel JP, Myers RH, Hedley-Whyte ET, *et al.* (1991). Cerebral amyloid angiopathy without and with cerebral hemorrhages: a comparative histological study. *Ann. Neurol.* **30**:637–649.

Wang X, Tsuji K, Lee SR, *et al.* (2004). Mechanisms of hemorrhagic transformation after tissue plasminogen activator reperfusion therapy for ischemic stroke. (Review) (50 refs) *Stroke* **35**(11 Suppl 1):2726–2730.

World Health Organization (1992). The ICD-10 Classification of Mental and Behavioural Disorders: Clinical Descriptions and Diagnostic Guidelines. World Health Organization, Geneva, Switzerland, pp. 50–51.

World Health Organization (1993). The ICD-10 Classification of Mental and Behavioural Disorders: Diagnostic Criteria for Research. World Health Organization, Geneva, Switzerland, pp. 36–40.

Zabramski JM, Henn JS, Coons S (1999). Pathology of cerebral vascular malformations. (Review) (92 refs) *Neurosurg. Clin. N. Am.* **10**:395–410.

Chapter 7

Dementia with Lewy bodies

Introduction

Largely unrecognized two decades ago, dementia with Lewy bodies (DLB) is now thought to be the second most common cause of dementia, accounting for 15–26% of cases at autopsy (McKeith *et al.*, 1996). DLB is one of a group of synucleinopathies (*Table 7.1*, overleaf) that are characterized by abnormal aggregation of the synaptic protein, alpha-synuclein. Other synucleinopathies include Parkinson's disease (PD), adult Hallervorden–Spatz disease, and multiple systems atrophy (MSA). Mutations in alpha-synuclein have been identified in familial PD (Polymeropoulos *et al.*, 1997; Vaughan *et al.*, 1998). While familial cases of DLB have been reported (Ohara *et al.*, 1999; Galvin *et al.*, 2002), no mutations have been identified in DLB as yet.

The clinical phenotype of DLB includes progressive dementia, extrapyramidal signs, visual hallucinations, and fluctuating cognitive status. DLB has had several diagnostic labels in the last decade, including diffuse Lewy-body disease, Lewy-body dementia, Lewy-body variant of Alzheimer's disease, and senile dementia of the Lewy-body type. Consensus guidelines were developed in 1996 to establish a common framework for the diagnosis and pathological assessment (McKeith *et al.*, 1996) (*Box 7.1*). These original diagnostic criteria have been revised and extended several times (McKeith *et al.*, 1999, 2005) (*Box 7.2*).

Box 7.1 Dementia with Lewy bodies 1996 Consensus criteria for the clinical diagnosis

- Dementia (required central feature):
  - Prominent memory impairment may not necessarily occur in the early stages but is usually evident with progression.
  - Deficits in attention, frontal-subcortical skills, and visuospatial abilities may be especially prominent.
- Two of the following core features must be present for a diagnosis of probable DLB, one for possible DLB:
  - Fluctuating cognition with pronounced variations in attention and alertness.
  - Recurrent visual hallucinations that are typically well formed and detailed.
  - Spontaneous motor features of parkinsonism.
- Features supportive of the diagnosis:
  - Repeated falls.
  - Syncope.
  - Transient loss of consciousness.
  - Neuroleptic sensitivity.
  - Systematized delusions.
  - Hallucinations in other modalities.
- A diagnosis of DLB is less likely in the presence of:
  - Stroke disease, evident as focal neurologic signs or on brain imaging.
  - Evidence on physical examination and investigation of any physical illness or other brain disorder sufficient to account for the picture.

(McKeith *et al.*, 1996)

Table 7.1 The major Lewy disorders (synucleinopathies)

Lewy disorder	Abnormal protein/s	Typical clinical features	Typical pathologic findings
PD[1] (No validated consensus criteria)	aSYN; ubiquitin	Early movement disorder: rigidity, bradykinesia, rest tremor, masked facies, en bloc turning, shuffling gait, and stooped posture	• Nigral pallor at autopsy • Nigral LBs, gliosis, and dopaminergic neuron loss • LN, aSYN lesions in neostriatum
DLB[2]	aSYN; ubiquitin	Dementia	• Brainstem LBs (nigra, LC, DMN) • Limbic LBs and LN (CA2/3, ERC, amygdala) • Neocortical LB (STG, anterior cingulate cortex)
Postencephalitic parkinsonism	aSYN; ubiquitin; tau	• Parkinsonism • Dementia • Hx 1918 viral encephalitis (variable)	• NFT (no SP) • Brainstem LB
MSA (MSA with GCI; form of spinocerebellar degeneration)	aSYN; ubiquitin	• Cerebellar ataxia • Parkinsonism • Dysautonomia • Dementia (variable)	
Motor neuron disorders (ALS, FTD-MND, Guamanian parkinsonism-ALS dementia complex)	aSYN; ubiquitin	• Dementia • Parkinsonism • Upper and lower motor symptoms • Nerve conduction slowed • Muscle group fiber atrophy; fasciculations	• Frontotemporal atrophy, neuron loss, gliosis in the absence of tauopathy pathology • aSYN+, ubiquitin+ inclusions anterior horn neurons, nigra
Hallervorden–Spatz disease (NBIA-I)	Iron (ferritin); aSYN; ubiquitin	• Dementia • Movement disorder	• Globus pallidus brown discoloration • Iron accumulation in globus pallidus • aSYN+ Lewy-like inclusions and LN in brainstem (nigra)
Familial Lewy dementia (DLB, PD, juvenile PD)	• PARK 1 (chromosome 4) • PARK 2 (chromosome 6) • PARK 3 (chromosome 2p13, 4p defined gene mutations)	• Early-onset PD or DLB, can be sole dementing disorder or co-occur with AD • Autosomal dominant for PARK 1,2,3 gene mutations on chromosomes 2,4,6	• Gene mutation • PD or DLB pathologic lesion pattern

[1]Mirra, 1991; [2]McKeith *et al.*, 1996
DMN: dorsal motor nucleus of the vagus cranial nerve (X); STG: superior temporal gyrus

Box 7.2 DLB Consortium Third Report: upgraded diagnosis and management criteria
- Added core features that suggest DLB:
  - REM sleep behavior disorder.
  - Severe neuroleptic sensitivity.
  - Reduced striatal dopamine transporter activity on functional neuroimaging.
- One year rule in differentiating DLB and PD dementia is less rigid:
  - May use Lewy body disease for ambiguous cases.
- New scheme for pathologic assessment:
  - aSYN immunohistochemistry replaces ubiquitin IHC for diagnosis.
  - Semiquantitative grading of Lewy bodies and Lewy neurites.
  - Lewy and Alzheimer pathology assigned probability rank as cause of DLB syndrome.
  - Regional lesion pattern more important than lesion amount.
- Management:
  - Improvements noted in attention, visual hallucinations, and sleep disorders with cholinesterase inhibitors.

(McKeith *et al.*, 1999; 2005)

Clinical features

The core clinical features of DLB include fluctuating cognitive impairment, recurrent visual hallucinations, and parkinsonism in the setting of dementia. The 1996 consensus criteria have been examined in several prospective studies (McKeith *et al.*, 2000; Lopez *et al.*, 2002). Overall, the criteria show a variable sensitivity ranging from 23% to 83% while specificity generally remains high (95–100%). There are ongoing efforts to improve the sensitivity of clinical criteria by enhancing consistent application and improving interrater reliability. These efforts are focusing on including more detailed definitions of the quality, frequency, and severity of core and supportive features (McKeith *et al.*, 2004).

Cognition
Individuals with DLB typically present with recurrent episodes of confusion on a background of progressive cognitive deterioration. The fluctuations in cognitive function are manifest as shifting attention and levels of alertness that may vary over minutes, hours, or days. The assessment of fluctuating cognitive impairment poses substantial difficulty to many clinicians. Four composite subtypes of fluctuating cognition have been shown to differentiate between DLB and AD: daytime drowsiness and lethargy, daytime sleep of 2+ hours, staring into space for long periods, and episodes of disorganized speech (Ferman *et al.*, 2004). Evidence of three (or more) of these feature composites was evident in 63% of DLB patients studied, as opposed to only 12% of AD patients and 0.5% of normal elderly individuals (*Box 7.3*, overleaf). Psychometric performance profiles are not part of the consensus criteria, although DLB patients tend to perform better on tests of verbal memory and worse on visuospatial performance tasks compared to individuals with AD.

Visual hallucinations
Psychiatric manifestations are common in DLB and predominantly consist of visual hallucinations (VH), delusions, apathy and anxiety. VH present early in the clinical course when dementia is relatively mild, and tend to persist. Typical VH in DLB are vivid, three-dimensional images of animate objects (e.g. children, animals). Visual hallucinations are associated with greater deficits in cortical acetylcholine and predict a better response to cholinesterase inhibitors.

Parkinsonism
Extrapyramidal signs develop in most DLB patients at some time in the course of the disease. Extrapyramidal signs, however, are not necessary for a clinical diagnosis of DLB; only 25–50% of DLB individuals have documented extrapyramidal dysfunction at the time of diagnosis. However, parkinsonism develops in the majority of affected individuals during the course of DLB. The extrapyramidal signs in DLB typically include postural instability, bradykinesia, and facial impassivity; tremor is less common.

Supportive features
Rapid eye movement (REM) sleep behavior disorders are frequently seen in DLB and other synucleinopathies such as PD and MSA. REM sleep behavior disorders are manifested as vivid or frightening dreams associated with simple or complex motor behavior. The presence of REM sleep behavior disorder is suggestive of DLB. Additionally,

Box 7.3 Dementia with Lewy bodies (DLB) *vs.* Alzheimer's disease (AD); a simplified clinical-neuropsychological comparison at the mild-moderate stage

Clinical profile	DLB	AD
Prevalence among dementias (%)	~20	~70
Common presenting complaints	Hallucinations, fluctuating inattention, visual distractibility	Forgetfulness
Neurologic/motor	Parkinsonism, frequent falls, syncope	Normal functioning
Neuropsychiatric	Visual hallucinations, auditory hallucinations, delusions	Depression, anxiety, delusions
Course from diagnosis to death	~6–10 years	~8–10 years
Progression	Fluctuating downward decline to global dementia	Gradual downward decline to global dementia

Neuropsychological profile	DLB	AD
Qualitative performance differences	Language interference (intrusions) and perseverative errors	Forgetfulness for instructions and receptive language problems
Confusion/disorientation	++	+
Attention/concentration deficits	+++	++
Episodic memory deficits	++	++++
Language deficits	++	++
Executive dysfunction	+++	+++
Visual–spatial deficits	++++	+
ADL impairment	+++	++

The '+' signs estimate relative impairment in a given cognitive-functional domain when assessed at the mild to moderate stage of disease progression. These estimates are based on neuropsychological profiles of typical/classic cases (see references below). It is important to recognize that clinical presentations of these disorders will vary, especially when mixed dementia pathologies are present.

(Ballard *et al.*, 2002; Doubleday *et al.*, 2002; Galvin, 2003; Noe *et al.*, 2003; McKeith *et al.*, 2004)

autonomic abnormalities are more common in DLB than in AD and include orthostatic hypotension and carotid sinus hypersensitivity. These abnormalities can result in 'dizziness', presyncope, syncope, and falls as common aspects of the clinical presentation.

Parkinson's disease dementia

Dementia is common in patients with PD, occurring in up to 40%. DLB and the dementia that occurs in PD have similar clinical and neuropathological phenotypes. Both DLB and PD dementia (PDD) are clinically defined syndromes. While validated consensus criteria exist for the clinical diagnosis of DLB, no formal consensus criteria exist for PDD. Currently, DLB and PDD are clinically distinguished using the arbitrary '1-year rule': PDD is diagnosed when the onset of dementia occurs 12 months or more after the onset of parkinsonism, otherwise by convention DLB is diagnosed.

The neuropathologic phenotype of DLB and PDD often are indistinguishable. Both PDD and DLB have Lewy bodies (LBs) present in the brainstem and cortex. PD is classically associated with the presence of LBs and neuron loss in the substantia nigra of the mid-brain, accounting for the predominant motor symptoms. In DLB, Lewy bodies are more widespread; in addition to being present in the brainstem they are found throughout the cerebral cortex, particularly the cingulum, insula, and temporal lobe, and in the transentorhinal allocortex. There are no definite pathologic criteria to separate PDD and DLB from each other or from PD without dementia. This aspect is discussed further in the Neuropathology section. It is possible that these syndromes are so similar at a biological level that a categorical distinction between DLB and PDD is inappropriate. The neuropathology of DLB is further complicated by significant overlap with AD pathology. Up to 91% of cases of DLB diagnosed pathologically have AD changes present with pure DLB accounting for a minority of cases (Hansen & Samuel, 1997). These indistinct neuropathological boundaries continue to be a source of nosological confusion and additional work will be necessary to resolve the issues.

Neuroimaging of DLB

Currently, neuroimaging is not part of the consensus clinical criteria for the diagnosis of DLB. In clinical practice, the current role of neuroimaging, as in the evaluation of any dementia, is to evaluate for the presence of alternate pathologies that may account for a decline in cognition (e.g. infarcts, tumor, hydrocephalus). Neuroimaging studies have demonstrated structural and functional differences between DLB and AD. Structural magnetic resonance imaging (MRI) scans in DLB patients generally reveal less temporal lobe and hippocampal atrophy early in the disease course compared to AD (Hashimoto et al., 1998; Barber et al., 1999, 2000) (7.1). DLB is associated with cerebral perfusion and metabolic changes in the occipital lobes using single photon emission computed tomography (SPECT) neuroimaging (Lobotesis et al., 2001), although gross structural changes in this region do not appear to occur (Middelkoop et al., 2001). Positron emission tomography (PET) studies show reduced dopamine receptor radio-chemical tracer signals in the neostriatum (caudate and putamen) in DLB compared to AD subjects (Hu et al., 2000), while structural changes in the putamen have been reported in DLB compared to AD, the basis of which may be the pathologic involvement of this area in the generation of extrapyramidal signs (Cousins et al., 2003). These findings suggest neuroimaging techniques may have the potential to augment the clinical diagnosis of DLB (*Box 7.4*).

7.1 Individuals with dementia with Lewy bodies (DLB) tend to have hippocampal volumes intermediate in size to nondemented individuals and individuals with Alzheimer's disease. (**A**) An 84-year-old nondemented male with full hippocampi bilaterally. (**B**) A 78-year-old female with DLB. The bilateral hippocampi are slightly atrophied, most evident by the enlarged temporal horns. (**C**) An 80-year-old male with very mild Alzheimer's disease and prominent hippocampal volume loss and severely enlarged temporal horns. Arrows denote hippocampi in all images.

Box 7.4 Emission tomography and SPECT in DLB

Dementing disorder	PET (metabolism)	SPECT (blood flow)
AD	Bilateral temporoparietal hypometabolism	Bilateral temporoparietal hypoperfusion
DLB	Reduced dopamine transporter (I-131)I-FP-CIT method	Medial parietal and occipital hypoperfusion
VaD – multi-infarct subtype	–	Multiple, asymmetric perfusion defects
VaD – subcortical subtype	Preserved oxygen extraction	Reduced perfusion
FTD	Frontotemporal lobar hypometabolism	Frontotemporal lobar hypoperfusion

AD, Alzheimer's disease; DLB, dementia with Lewy bodies; VaD, vascular dementia; FTD, frontotemporal dementia. (Pakrasi & O'Brien, 2005)

Neuropathology of Lewy body disorders

This family of neurodegenerative disorders has in common: (1) a molecular abnormality in the synapse-associated protein alpha-synuclein (aSYN); (2) the pathologic burden can be grouped as brainstem, limbic, and neocortical forms of Lewy disease; and (3) core pathologic features are the presence of classical Lewy bodies, pigmented neuron loss and gliosis in the substantia nigra (SN) and locus ceruleus (LC), CA 2/3 neurites, and aSYN-positive Lewy neurites (LN). Superimposed on these core histologic features are various lesions that morphologically define specific clinicopathologic disease entities classified within the broader Lewy spectrum of neurologic diseases. *Table 7.1* presents the currently recognized major types of DLB.

7.2 On the left are hemicoronal sections through the mid-brain and substantia nigra (top) and the pons and LC (bottom) of a PD brainstem (sections at left) and an AD brainstem (sections at right). The midline of all sections is to the right. The lateral portion of the PD nigra is more depigmented and appears pale compared to the uniformly black AD nigra. The LC of the PD brain is severely depigmented and is barely visible compared to the black LC of the AD brain bordering and to the left of the cerebral aqueduct. (Formalin fixed autopsy specimen.)

Parkinson's disease

This is the prototypic disease among the Lewy body (synucleinopathy) family of biochemically related disorders. Sir James Parkinson described 'An essay on the shaking palsy' in 1817. Frederick Lewy (1912, 1913) first described the inclusions that bear his name in the hypothalamus and drew no connection of clinical parkinsonism to nigral inclusions. Subsequently, classic Lewy bodies, astrocytic gliosis, and severe depletion of SN pigmented dopaminergic neurons were identified as the triad that best identified cases of clinical PD (Hughes *et al.*, 1993a, b; Forno, 1996).

The SN shows lateral severe pallor in typical motor PD that contrasts with the deep black pigment of normal control brains or the often well preserved pigment of AD brains (7.2). Demented PD patients also have medial SN and ventral tegmental area (VTA) pallor (Rinne *et al.*, 1989). Hematoxylin eosin (H&E) preparations of the SN show marked neuron loss, gliosis, and increased free neuromelanin pigment (7.3–7.5). Classical nigral Lewy bodies may be visualized with H&E (7.6), or ubiquitin (7.7) or aSYN (7.8, 7.9) immunohistochemistry (*Box 7.5*).

7.3 The substantia nigra pars compacta of a pure DLB case reveals mild neuronal depletion, gliosis, and free neuromelanin deposits in the neuropil (two circled areas). A classic LB (black arrow) and two dopaminergic neurons with pale bodies (yellow arrows) are also evident. (H&E ×10 objective.)

7.4 The classical triad of nigral lesions that define idiopathic PD pathology: **A**: Free neuromelanin in the neuropil and within macrophages, with localized gliosis marked by crowded small glial nuclei; **B**: A classical intraneuronal haloed LB; **C**: A pale body LB precursor. **D**: A typical CLB in the cytoplasm of the lower neuron. (H&E, ×40 objective.)

7.5 Free neuromelanin brown pigment in the neuropil and within cerebral macrophages surrounding LB remnants marks the site of degenerated dopaminergic neurons in the SN pars compacta of a PD patient. **A**: H&E appearance of pigment-containing cells clustered around a naked LB core; **B**: Free and cytoplasmic neuromelanin surrounding a partly digested LB core that has been labeled with aSYN LB-509 antibody (blue substrate). (Both panels, ×40 objective.)

7.6 Typical diagnostic H&E profile of classical nigral LBs in PD. **A**: The brown cytoplasmic neuromelanin pigment of a large nigral dopaminergic neuron is displaced to form an irregularly contoured pale body at the center and upper right of the soma. A small classical LB occupies the 9 o'clock position next to the outer cellular membrane and just above the cell nucleus; **B**: A normal pars compacta nigral dopaminergic neuron is positioned below a pigmented neuron with a pyknotic dark nucleus and a circular classical LB with a lamellar substructure that displaces the cytoplasmic neuromelanin. The surrounding neuropil is gliotic. (H&E both panels, ×40 objective.)

7.7 Anterior cingulate cortex of a DLB brain has been immunostained with polyvalent antibody to ubiquitin (DAB brown substrate). The medium sized neuron at upper right contains a typical, cytoplasmic, round to angular CLB. The smallest ubiquinated structures in the neuropil may represent cross-sectioned dendrites, while the largest structure could be either an extracellular LB (less likely) or a corpora amylacea (more likely). (Ubiquitin-DAB immunohistochemistry, ×40 objective.)

7.8 A composite illustrates five types of LB inclusions in nigral dopaminergic neurons of a pure DLB patient. **A, B**: Reticulated aSYN LBs within cytoplasmic pools of nondisplaced neuromelanin; **C**: A torpedo-shaped giant meganeurite that is as large as the neuronal cell nucleus in **D**. The cytoplasm of the latter neuron contains a minute grape-like aSYN deposit. The cytoplasm of neurons in **A–E** also contains fine granular aSYN deposits; **E**: Dumbbell-shaped classic LB with strong rim enhancement and a clearer center. A circular single-lobed classical LB is illustrated in **F**. Segments of fine LNs may be seen in **A, B, E**, and **F**. (Anti-aSYN antibody LB-509 and a dark blue substrate with nuclear fast red counterstain, ×40 objective.)

7.9 Two nigral dopaminergic neurons contain almost circular pale bodies that are eosinophilic and appear to be clear of other cytoplasmic elements. The remainder of the cytoplasm is occupied by blue Nissl substance (primarily rough endoplasmic reticulum) and fine brown neuromelanin granules. (H&E, ×40 objective.)

Box 7.5 Immunohistochemistry of pale and Lewy bodies: labeling with anti-ubiquitin antibodies

A: Pale bodies and classical Lewy bodies by H&E in dopaminergic pigmented neurons of the substantia nigra. Lewy bodies have a dense, strongly eosinophilic central core that is surrounded by a clear halo. Pale bodies are intracytoplasmic precursor lesions to mature Lewy bodies. Clear palely eosinophilic material displaces neuromelanin granules. Both classical Lewy body cores (**B**) and entire pale bodies (**C**) label strongly with a polyvalent ubiquitin-specific antiserum. A similar pattern would be evident using monoclonal antibodies to alpha-synuclein (not shown here).

7.10 Caudal SN of a DLB brainstem displays copious thin and coarse LN in various spatial orientations surrounding dopaminergic neuromelanin-containing neurons with aSYN immunoreactive focal deposits (neuron at left), a cluster of free neuromelanin pigment (below left neuron), and two fused LBs (neuron at right). (aSYN immunohistochemistry, blue substrate, ×40 objective.)

7.11 Two LC probable noradrenergic neurons from a pure DLB brain display aSYN immunoreactive inclusions plus diffuse punctate immunoreactivity throughout the cytoplasm. Synaptic immunoreactivity has been suppressed with protease 24 pretreatment of the section. The surrounding neuropil contains fine to coarse LNs, some of which end in expanded boutons while others exhibit segmental swellings ('beading'). (6 μm paraffin section, aSYN LB-509 monoclonal antibody, blue substrate, P24 pretreatment, ×40 objective.)

7.12 A classic LB of the type first described by FH Lewy is shown in a magnocellular, probable cholinergic, neuron of the NBM from a pure DLB case. Periinclusion cytoplasmic clearing and a faintly spiculated outer boundary of the LB core are evident. (H&E, ×40 objective.)

7.13 A small classical haloed LB (arrow) is seen in one of four magnocellular NBM neurons in a mixed AD–DLB case. (H&E, ×40 objective.)

7.14 An axonal spheroid appears as a spherical structure that lacks a nucleus but includes eosinophilic to basophilic granular elements. Such structures may be occasionally encountered in PD or DLB in the SN. They occur in a much more widespread distribution and in larger numbers in Hallervorden–Spatz disease. (H&E, ×40 objective.)

LBs are frequently circular in shape and the core outer boundary is surrounded by spicules and a halo that separates the core from the surrounding cytoplasm and brown neuromelanin pigment (Gomez-Tortosa *et al.*, 2000). Electron microscopy of LBs shows a finely fibrillar substructure (Arima *et al.*, 1998). The immunostaining methods also reveal both fine and thick meganeurites (**7.10**) in the same regions where classical haloed LBs are most frequent: the SN *pars compacta* (mid-brain), the LC (upper pons) (**7.11**), and the nucleus basalis of Meynert (NBM) (**7.12**, **7.13**). Lewy first described LBs in the NBM (1912, 1913). Corpora amylacea (see **4.4**) and axonal spheroids (**7.14**) in the same anatomic regions should not be confused with LBs.

H&E does not reveal changes in the caudate and putamen (neostriatum), despite biochemical and *in vivo* imaging evidence that striatal dopamine receptors are depleted. Novel antibodies have been developed that demonstrate abundant lesions in neostriatal structures in addition to SN and LC (Miller *et al.*, 1999; Duda *et al.*, 2002). Newer histochemical, silver-based methods (Braak & Braak, 1999; Sandmann-Keil *et al.*, 1999; Hishikawa *et al.*, 2001) and

---

Box 7.6: Lesion progression in Parkinson's disease (PD)

Earliest anatomic lesions (presymptomatic stages 1 and 2)
• Medulla oblongata:
  – Glossopharyngeal-vagus nerve complex (brainstem)
  – Projection neurons of the intermediate reticular zone
  – Hypoglossal nerve nucleus (brainstem)
• Anterior olfactory nucleus
• Olfactory bulb and tract

Brainstem and basal forebrain lesions (overt clinical stages 3 and 4)
• Substantia nigra (mid-brain)
• Ceruleus-subceruleus complex (pons)
• Caudal raphe nuclei
• Gigantocellular reticular nucleus
• Basal forebrain and limbic areas:
  – Amygdala
  – Entorhinal allocortex
  – Nucleus basalis of Meynert

Telencephalic cortical lesions (end-stages 5 and 6)
• Anteriomedial temporal mesocortex
• Higher order sensory and prefrontal areas
• Other cortical areas

(Del Tredici *et al.*, 2002; Braak *et al.*, 2002, 2003)

---

nucleic acid, slide-based probes (Nisbet *et al.*, 1996; Eve *et al.*, 1997; Cannizzaro *et al.*, 2003) have been developed for the same purpose.

There is growing appreciation that Lewy lesions start and progress in a hierarchical pattern reminiscent of AD pathology (Jellinger, 1991; Del Tredici *et al.*, 2002; Braak *et al.*, 2003; Jellinger & Mizuno, 2003) (*Box 7.6*). The basal forebrain *anterior olfactory nucleus* and *dorsal motor nucleus of the vagus* in the medulla are early target neurons of aSYN immunopositive LBs and neurites.

Dementia with Lewy bodies

Grossly, the brain of a DLB patient with little or no AD pathology exhibits less overall cortical and hippocampal atrophy compared to a pure AD brain from a person with a similar degree of dementia severity. The sectioned SN in DLB is usually not as pale as in idiopathic PD (IPD) or in PDD, nor is the degree of neuron loss, gliosis, and free neuromelanin as substantial. The DLB SN usually is at least mildly to moderately pale compared to the SN of a brain from a nondemented control of similar age (**7.15**). The latter observation coincides with the less prevalent motor symptoms in pure DLB patients, and to their diminished responsivity to L-dopa therapy, compared to IPD patients.

The microscopic features of pure DLB include the following lesions: (1) presence of some classic LBs in either or both of SN and LC; (2) the presence of widespread, ubiquitin and aSYN immunoreactive cortical type LBs (CLBs) in selected hippocampal, limbic, and cortical regions (**7.16**, **7.17**); and (3) widespread occurrence in cortex, limbic, and brainstem areas of aSYN containing

dystrophic or LNs (**7.18**). CLBs typically are found in the superior temporal gyrus, anterior cingulate cortex, insular cortex, entorhinal cortex layer V (**7.19**), in the transitional allocortex along the descending limb of the collateral sulcus (**7.20**), the NBM (**7.12**, **7.13**), and the amygdala (**7.21**, **7.22**).

A special group of LNs occurs in the CA2/1 junctional region, where the narrow CA2 region widens into the CA1 subfield of the hippocampus (Dickson *et al.*, 1994) (**7.23**). Note the original publication refers to this as region 'CA2/3' because the primary hippocampal subfield affected is CA2 with some extension into both CA3 and CA1 subfields. The CA2/1 junctional region also first develops neuropil threads in AD before the entire CA1 region becomes widely involved with neurofibrillary pathology (see Chapter 5).

A minor subset of classical Lewy bodies may stain with tau antibody immunohistochemistry (**7.24**) or the modified Bielschowsky silver method (**7.25**). A large majority of LBs are negative with these stains in the authors' hands.

7.15 The normally pigmented SN of a nondemented 75-year-old woman (**A**) is contrasted with the moderate depigmentation of a 70-year-woman with mixed AD and PD of 21 years duration (**B**). Sections are at the level of the red nucleus (**B**, left) and the oculomotor cranial nerve nucleus (**A** and **B**, right). (Formalin fixed autopsy brainstem specimen.)

7.16 The six panels show typical CLBs from different DLB brains as displayed in routine 6 μm thick paraffin histologic sections. CLB shapes vary from circular to oval. No well defined halos are seen, however the CLBs in the far left and right upper panels and the far right lower panel do have central more dense regions. (H&E, ×40 objective.)

7.17 A–H: Typical CLBs immunostained by aSYN monoclonal antibody LB-509. **D** shows a similar medium-sized neuron that lacks a CLB for comparison. CLB shapes vary from circular to oval to bi-lobed (**B**). Blue minute puncta in the neuropil represent individual synapses. (aSYN, blue substrate, no protease pretreatment, ×40 objective.)

7.18 A composite array of aSYN immunoreactive pathologic structures from various brain regions in DLB cases. Lesions include: fine, coarse, bouton-bearing, and mega-LNs; reticular and compact cytoplasmic Lewy inclusions and rim-enhancing LBs; free neuromelanin in neuropil; and an aSYN-IR torpedo at far lower right. (aSYN LB-509, blue substrate, ×40 objective.)

7.19 CLBs in four brain regions of DLB cases: **A**: Superior temporal gyrus cortex; **B**: Anterior cingulate cortex; **C**: Insula; **D**: ERC IV/V. CLBs in **A** and **C** are circular, whereas those in panels **B** and **D** are irregular with indentations (**B**) or excavations along the surface (**D**). (**A**, **B**, and **D**: aSYN with blue substrate, nuclear fast red counterstain, ×40 objective; **C**: H&E, ×40 objective.)

7.20 Two circular dense cortical LBs from an AD–DLB case (AD–LB variant) co-exist with fine LNs in transitional allocortex bordering the medial bank of the collateral sulcus. (aSYN, ×40 objective.)

7.21 The medial and basal amygdala of pure or mixed DLB cases often contain a massive meshwork of CLBs and ramifying LNs. (aSYN immunostain, ×20 objective.)

7.22 H&E appearance of amygdalar (**A**) and entorhinal (amygdala level) (**B**) CLBs in pure DLB.

7.23 LNs often occur in DLB brains at the junction of hippocampal pyramidal layer cellular regions CA2 and CA1, where the former first widens out progressing laterally. Some LNs may extend to involve CA3 as well. This anatomic pattern has been referred to as 'CA2/3 neurites'. (aSYN immunostaining, ×20 objective.)

7.24 A subset of otherwise histologically typical LBs may immunostain positively with antibodies that are specifically directed to phosphorylated tau epitopes. **A**: A nigral dopaminergic pigmented neuron with two LBs (1) that have tau-positive cores. In contrast, pale bodies are weakly stained or unstained (2); **B**: Two similar tau-immunoreactive LBs (1, 2). (PHF-1 monoclonal antibody directed to hyperphosphorylated tau epitopes at serine 396 and 404 [gift of Peter Davies], DAB substrate, ×40 objective.)

7.25 The central core of a nigral classical LB in a DLB case stains robustly with the modified Bielschowsky silver impregnation method. Such a finding is distinctly unusual in the author's experience. The black intensely argyrophilic material in the neuronal cytoplasm is neuromelanin. (mBT silver stain, ×40 objective.)

The diagnostic dilemma of Parkinsonian syndrome with dementia

Patients with classical PD form a subset of patients with parkinsonian symptoms. From the pathologist's point of view at autopsy the major disorders that are associated with parkinsonian dementia are AD with extrapyramidal symptoms (Burns *et al.*, 2005), mixed PD with AD pathology (the so-called LB variant of AD) (Hansen *et al.*, 1990) (**7.26**), and pure LB disease. The latter may represent end-stage PD that has progressed to diffuse LB disease, or DLB from the outset. The two latter conditions may be distinguished primarily by observing more macroscopic pallor and greater dopaminergic neuron loss in the SN in long-standing motor PD. The SN may not be severely depigmented in a significant proportion of pure DLB cases.

Postencephalitic Parkinsonism

Drs Evidente and Gwinn of the Mayo Clinic (1998) offer the following clinical description of the disorder:

'Encephalitis lethargica, also known as von Economo's encephalitis, was a global pandemic that affected more than a million people all over the world from 1915 to 1930. Although parkinsonism was occasionally seen during the acute encephalitic phase of encephalitis lethargica, it was often encountered in the postencephalitic phase. The onset of postencephalitic parkinsonism can be delayed by several years from the resolution of encephalitis lethargica'.

The gross and microscopic pathologic features are similar to those of ordinary idiopathic PD (IPD) with one notable

7.26 The admixture of Alzheimer NFTs (**A**) and neuritic NPs (**B**) with anterior cingulate gyrus CLBs and neurites (**C**) and entorhinal CLBs and fine LNs at the amygdalar level (**D**) is illustrated for a mixed AD (Braak stage VI-C) and DLB 1996 consensus criteria neocortical type case. (**A, B**: Modified Bielschowsky silver method, ×40 objective; **C, D**: aSYN LB-509 antibody immunostaining with ×10 objective [**C**] and ×40 objective [**D**]).

exception (Gibb & Lees, 1987): that is, in addition to LBs, Alzheimer neurofibrillary tangles (NFTs) are widespread in the absence of widespread senile plaques that typify AD (Wong *et al.*, 1996). The exact etiology and viral nature of this disorder remains controversial despite recent probe analysis of DNA from archival brain specimens (Hudson & Rice, 1990; Jellinger, 2001).

Familial Lewy disorders

The spectrum of hereditary parkinsonian syndromes is rapidly expanding with the advent of increasingly broad genomic screening. At present, mutations in only two genes have been demonstrated to cause disorders that mimic young and mature onset IPD but not DLB: (1) the *alpha-synuclein* gene; and (2) the *parkin* gene. The pathology of IPD dementia and DLB exhibits marked overlap as discussed earlier in the chapter (*Box 7.7*). Some but not all *parkin* gene mutations are associated with LB inclusions even though there is usually severe degeneration of the SN pars compacta. Other genes that are currently implicated in causing adult parkinsonism include *DJ-1* (Bonifati *et al.*, 2003), *PINK-1* (Valente *et al.*, 2004), *LRRK2* that specifies the protein *dardarin* (Paisin-Ruiz *et al.*, 2005), *UHC-L1* (ubiquitin C-terminal hydrolase isozyme L1) (Snyder & Wolozin, 2004), and nuclear receptor-related factor 1 (*Boxes 7.8, 7.9*).

Juvenile PD

By definition, juvenile PD begins before age 21 years and leads to typical parkinsonian signs and symptoms. Most cases are now recognized to be associated with mutations in the *parkin* gene (AR-JP, PARK2, Parkin gene, OMIM #602544) (*Box 7.8*) (Clarimon *et al.*, 2005). Only a single case has been described with typical LBs (Yoshimura *et al.*, 1988), thus age may be a permissive factor for Lewy formation. This would be consistent with observations that incidental (preclinical) LB disease is sharply age-associated (Forno, 1969). In 273 brains, age-specific prevalence of LBs increased from 3.8% to 12.8% between the sixth and ninth decades (Gibb & Lees, 1988).

Familial DLB

A number of pedigrees have been described in which the presentation resembles spontaneous DLB (Galvin *et al.*, 2002). LB pathology may be the sole dementia substrate or may occur with Alzheimer plaques and tangles, the so-called AD Lewy body variant (Ohara *et al.*, 1999; Galvin *et al.*, 2002) (**7.25**). As in cases of spontaneous DLB, the density of CLBs bears same relationship to the severity of clinical dementia. In mixed AD–DLB, the combined pathologies seem to have an additive or synergistic effect. Gearing *et al.* (1999) have demonstrated two types of mixed AD–DLB pathology, the low- and high-tangle variants.

Box 7.7 Genetics of Lewy disorders

Familial Parkinson's disease (PD) gene mutations that have Lewy bodies[1]

- aSYN (multiple missense and genomic multiplication mutations including A53T and A30P, E46K)[2,3,4]
- Nuclear receptor-related 1 (Nurr1)[7,8]
- Locus on chromosome 2[3]

Ubiquitin-proteasome system mutations (atypical PD not associated with Lewy bodies)

- Parkin gene (8 subtypes):
  - PARK 1[5] on long arm of chromosome 4
  - PARK 2[5] chromosome 6 – autosomal recessive juvenile
  - PARK 3[5] chromosome 2p13
  - Chromosome 4p[5]
  - Ubiquitin C-terminal hydroxylase L1 (UCHL1)
  - DJ-1/PARK7[6] molecular chaperone to aSYN

Candidate genes that have been screened with no definite mutations

- Dopamine cell survival
- Dopamine synthesis, metabolism, and function
- Energy supply
- Oxidative stress
- Cellular detoxification

[1]Huang *et al.*, 2004; [2]Pals *et al.*, 2004; [3]Ramsden *et al.*, 2001; [4]Choi *et al.*, 2004; [5]Gasser, 2000; [6]Bonifati *et al.*, 2003; [7]Conway *et al.*, 1998; [8]Ramsden *et al.*, 2001.

Box 7.8 Gene locations in Parkinson's disease

Name of mutation	Age of onset (years)	Mutated gene and chromosome location	Lewy body presence
PARK 1	Younger than spontaneous PD	*aSYN*, chr.4, Ala53Thr, Ala30Pro	Yes; Contoursi kindred with tau
PARK 2	<40	*parkin*, long arm Chr.6, exonic deletions and point mutations	No, severe SN degeneration
PARK 3	–	Chr.2	No, SN + LC degeneration
PARK 4	25–48	Chr.4, short arm	Yes, resembles DLB
PARK 5	–	Chr.1 short arm, near PARK 5	–
PARK 6	Wide range	Chr.1 short arm	–
PARK 7	–	Chr.1 (DJ-1) short arm, near PARK 6	–
PARK 8	38–68	Chr.12q11.2-p13.1	No, SN degeneration
PARK 10	Late onset	–	–
UCH-L1	–	Chr.4 short arm, Lie93Met, Ubiquitin carboxyterminal hydrolase-L1 enzyme reduced to 50% of normal	–

chr.: chromosome; DLB: dementia with Lewy bodies; IPD: idiopathic Parkinson's disease; LC: locus ceruleus; SN: substantia nigra; –: information not known.
(Jellinger *et al.*, 2003)

Box 7.9 Familial Parkinson's disease gene penetrance
Autosomal dominant genes
- *aSYN*
- *LRRK-2* (dardarin)

Autosomal recessive genes
- *parkin*
- *PINK-1*
- *DJ-1*

(Morris, 2005)

Both autosomal dominant and recessive patterns of inheritance have been documented. An issue here is the difficulty in distinguishing between familial idiopathic PD and DLB. In the former, as discussed in the preceding sections, numerous mutations in various *parkin* gene phenotypes have been published. For pure DLB *per se*, to date no point mutations have been described in the literature.

Vascular parkinsonism

Some cases of parkinsonism have a vascular etiology (VPD), as originally described by Critchley in 1929 (see Sibon *et al.*, 2004; Sibon & Tison, 2004 for recent reviews). The clinical profiles for VPD differ from spontaneous idiopathic PD (sIPD) in having more vascular risk factors, infrequent resting tremor, and a less frequent favorable response to L-dopa medication (15% for VaPD *vs.* 90% for sIPD) (Rampello *et al.*, 2005; Thanvi *et al.*, 2005; Turnbull, 2005). Neuroimaging modalities including SPECT (Lorberboym *et al.*, 2004), PET (Nurmi *et al.*, 2001), and MRI (Zijlmans *et al.*, 1995) brain scans may provide useful discrimination between vascular and nonvascular etiologies of PD.

Typical PD lesions such as LBs and LNs are absent on histologic examination. Several types of vascular pathology have been described as the basis for VPD (Zjlmans *et al.*, 2004). Striatal, nigral, and large territorial infarcts (~15% of cases) are rarely associated with VPD. Common underlying lesions include evidence of multiple subcortical lacunar infarcts that interrupt thalamocortical neural fiber pathways, and evidence of small vessel disease. The latter lesions include microscopic perivascular pallor by H&E and LFB-PAS, hyaline thickening of blood vessels walls, and dilated Virchow–Robins spaces.

Box 7.10 Multiple system atrophy (MSA)
Clinical features
- Parkinsonism (90%), 50% with cerebellar or pyramidal features
- Cerebellar and pyramidal signs:
- 80% MSA-P (striatonigral) (30% with, 50% without, cerebellar features)
- 20% MSA-C (olivopontocerebellar atrophy) (10% with, 10% without, parkinsonism)
- Autonomic failure (90%) 50% with cerebellar or pyramidal features

Pathology
- Cerebral and cerebellar (MSA-C) atrophy
- GCI (glial cell or Papp-Lantos inclusions): Gallyas silver+, ubiquitin+, aSYN+, tau+ (white matter >gray matter)
- Neuronal loss, astrocytosis, loss of myelin, microglial activation in substantia nigra, locus ceruleus, putamen, inferior olives, pontine nuclei, Purkinje cells, intermediolateral cell columns of the spinal cord
- Lewy bodies: not characteristic

(Kume *et al.*, 1991; Colisimo *et al.*, 1995; Spargo *et al.*, 1996; Inoue *et al.*, 1997; Gilman *et al.*, 1999; Dickson *et al.*, 1999; Lantos *et al.*, 2003)

Multiple system atrophy

The clinical features, including diagnostic criteria formulated by the North American MSA Study Group, are described in *Boxes 7.10, 7.11*. Ozawa *et al.* (2004) found that 34% of the cases were striatonigral (SND-), and 17% were olivopontocerebellar ataxia (OPCA)-predominant, terms that are based on pathologic findings, while the remainder (49%) had equivalent SND and OPCA pathology. Recent consensus criteria recommend that patients with predominantly parkinsonian features should be designated MSA-P, whereas those with predominantly cerebellar features are designated MSA-C (Wenning *et al.*, 1994; Burn & Jaros, 2001; Lantos & Quinn, 2003).

This disorder is linked to IPD and DLB primarily because the pathognomonic inclusions, the oligodendroglial *glial cell inclusions* (GCI), contain aSYN (**7.27A**) (Tu *et al.*, 1998) and ubiquitin immunoreactivity (*Box 7.12*). GCI also

Box 7.11 Multiple system atrophy (MSA): (North American Study Group)

Clinical features
- 12 US centers, 87 patients enrolled in first year
- Most with parkinsonian features
- Lasting asymmetry common
- One-third L-dopa responsive with common complications
- Two-thirds cerebellar dysfunction, of these 90% ataxic
- Urinary incontinence common
- Sleep disorder in most (rapid eye movement sleep behavior disorder and obstructive sleep apnea)

Neuroradiological features: SPECT
- Technetium-99 (ECD-SPECT) compared: 36 MSA, 43 PD, and 39 age-matched controls
- Dopamine transporter imaging overlap MSA and PD
- D2 dopamine receptor (IBZM marker) overlap MSA and PD
- ECD-SPECT reduced in striatum, cerebellum and brainstem in MSA compared to PD

PD: Parkinson's disease
(Gilman et al., 2005; Cilia et al., 2005)

Box 7.12 Differential staining of Lewy bodies and giant cell inclusions in multiple system atrophy (MSA)

Labeling method	GCI in MSA	Lewy body
aSYN IHC[1]	Strongly & variably positive	Strongly positive
Ubiquitin IHC[1]	Strongly positive	Strongly positive
Thiazin red fluorescent dye[1]	Consistently negative	Weakly positive or negative
Gallyas–Braak silver[1,2]	Positive	Negative
Campbell–Switzer method[2]	Positive	Positive
Tau IHC[3]	Rare subset positive nonphosphorylated >phosphorylated antibodies	Minor subset positive

GCI: glial cell inclusion; IHC: immunohistochemistry
[1]Sakamoto et al., 2005; [2]Uchihara et al., 2005; [3]Giasson et al., 2003

7.27 A: Diagnostic brainstem (oligodendroglial primarily) GCI in the WM from a case of adult MSA demonstrated with the LB-509 aSYN immunostaining technique. Note the shape of GCI with sharp spikes and hooks. (aSYN, nuclear fast red counterstain, ×40 objective.) **B**: Oligodendroglial GCI have been stained by the Gallyas silver method and have a similar appearance to their aSYN immunostained counterparts shown in **A**. (Gallyas silver method, ×40 objective.)

stain robustly with the Gallyas silver method (**7.27B**). They are negative or rarely positive with modified Bielschowsky silver methods or thiazin red (a NFT marker) (Kobayashi *et al.*, 1992; Cairns *et al.*, 1997; Giasson *et al.*, 2003). GCI immunolabel with nonphosphorylation-dependent tau antibodies in a rare subset of some MSA cases only. Most GCI are tau-immunonegative, based on the literature and personal experience. Tau epitopes may co-occur with 14-3-3 protein in GCI (*Box 7.12*). White matter contains many more GCI than gray matter, and GCI tend to accumulate preferentially in certain cortical laminae (Armstrong *et al.*, 2005). GCI concentrate in the posterior cerebrum and brainstem, especially in the mid-brain and pons, as shown in **7.27**.

Hallervorden–Spatz (H-S) or neurodegeneration with brain iron deposition, type 1 (NBIA-I)

Both childhood and adult forms are recognized (Racette *et al.*, 2001; Thomas *et al.*, 2004). Recent genetic breakthroughs have identified a mutation in the pantothenate kinase 2 (*PANK2*) gene on chromosome 20p12.3-p13 in some affected pedigrees (Zhou *et al.*, 2001). The adult form of H-S/NBIA-1 mainfests grossly as an atrophic brain with abnormally brown or brown-gray globus pallidus due to iron accumulation, seen when the brain is sectioned (Hayflick *et al.*, 2003; Jellinger & Duda, 2003; Baumeister *et al.*, 2005). Autopsy studies link NBIA-1 to other Lewy disorders by demonstrating widespread neuronal aSYN pathology (Arawaka *et al.*, 1998; Wakabayashi *et al.*, 1999; Galvin *et al.*, 2000; Jellinger *et al.*, 2003), including LBs and LNs, in the pallido-nigral system and red nucleus. NFTs are rare and may be age-associated. Major lesions are accumulation of iron-containing pigment (with neuromelanin and lipofuscin) in neurons, astrocytes, spheroids, microglia, free in the neuropil and around small vessels, and demyelination (status dysmyelinisatus). Later lesions include neuron loss, astrogliosis, spheroids predominately in medial globus pallidus and SN *pars reticulata*. Spheroids also occur in the subthalamic nucleus, striatum (caudate and putamen), thalamus, brainstem tegmentum, and nigra (**7.14**), cerebral cortex and spinal cord. Beta-synuclein and gamma-synuclein pathology has been demonstrated in three cases of NBIA-1 in distinctive neuronal and glial cell cytoplasmic inclusions and dystrophic neurites (Galvin *et al.*, 2000). Lesions in skeletal muscle, liver, bone marrow, and pituitary in NBIA-1 have been described in the literature (Galvin *et al.*, 2000).

7.28 Three anterior horn spinal cord motor neurons from a FTD-MND case exhibit Lewy-like round, sharply delineated Lewy-like inclusions that stain with ubiquitin polyvalent specific antiserum. (Anti-ubiquitin polyvalent antibody, DAB substrate immunostaining, ×40 objective.)

Motor neuron disease

The clinical features of this family of disorders are described in Chapter 8. Classical amyotrophic lateral sclerosis (ALS) patients may exhibit ubiquinated, aSYN-positive inclusions that resemble classical LBs in spinal cord anterior horn cells and in certain brainstem neuronal nuclei (Kato *et al.*, 1999). Another set of cases are thought to represent frontotemporal dementia with some features of motor neuron disease (FTD-MND). Gross skeletal muscle atrophy and microscopic group fiber atrophy on biopsy or at autopsy are usually far less severe than in classic ALS. FTD-MND cases may also have ubiquitinated anterior horn cell and cortical plus dentate fascia cytoplasmic Lewy-like inclusions (**7.28**). FTD-MND is discussed further as an entity in Chapter 8.

Surgical complications of treating Lewy body diseases

The scope of this monograph did not include medical treatment for dementing disorders. Surgical approaches may now be used to control some of the disabling motor symptoms of PD and DLB by interrupting specifically related neural pathways. Figure **7.29** illustrates a fortunately rare surgical complication of internal globus pallidus ablation ('pallidectomy'). The application of such surgical techniques reflects another example of our ever increasing knowledge base of basic disease pathophysiology within this important group of disorders.

7.29 A rare complication of surgical pallidectomy to alleviate the motor symptoms of PD is illustrated in this coronal brain section at the level of the mammillary bodies. The patient underwent surgical ablation of the medial globus pallidus 9 months prior to his death. At autopsy, pathologic residua of an old perioperative hematoma were found along the path of the electrode tract. Hemorrhage and cystic infarction involve the left caudate, putamen, and inner and outer globus pallidus, apparently sparing the left hypothalamus. The left frontal horn is narrowed by the swollen basal ganglia. The temporal horns are approximately equal in size. (Formalin fixed autopsy specimen.)

References

Aarawaka S, Saito Y, Murayama S, Mori H (1998). Lewy body in neurodegeneration with brain iron accumulation type 1 is immunoreactive for alpha-synuclein. *Neurology* **51**:887–889.

Arima K, Ueda K, Sunohara N, *et al.* (1998). Immunoelectron-microscopic demonstration of NACP/alpha-synuclein-epitopes on the filamentous component of Lewy bodies in Parkinson's disease and in dementia with Lewy bodies. *Brain Res.* **808**:93–100.

Armstrong RA. Lantos PL. Cairns NJ (2005). Multiple system atrophy: laminar distribution of the pathological changes in frontal and temporal neocortex: a study in ten patients. *Clin. Neuropathol.* **24**:230–235.

Ballard CG, Aarsland D, McKeith I *et al.* (2002). Fluctuations in attention: PD dementia vs. DLB with parkinsonism. *Neurology* **59**(11):1714–1720.

Barber R, Ballard C, McKeith IG, *et al.* (2000). MRI volumetric study of dementia with Lewy bodies: a comparison with AD and vascular dementia. *Neurology* **54**:1304–1309.

Barber R, Gholkar A, Scheltens P, *et al.* (1999). Medial temporal lobe atrophy on MRI in dementia with Lewy bodies. *Neurology* **52**:1153–1158.

Baumeister FA, Auer DP, Hortnagel K, *et al.* (2005). The eye-of-the-tiger sign is not a reliable disease marker for Hallervorden–Spatz syndrome. *Neuropediatrics* **36**:221–222.

Bonifati V, Rizzu P, van Baren MJ, *et al.* (2003). Mutations in the DJ-1 gene associated with autosomal recessive early-onset parkinsonism. *Science* **299**:256–259.

Burns JM, Galvin J, Roe CM, *et al.* (2005). The substantia nigra in Alzheimer's disease with extrapyramidal signs. *Neurology* **64**:1397–1403.

Braak E, Braak H (1999). Silver staining method for demonstrating Lewy bodies in Parkinson's disease and argyrophilic oligodendrocytes in multiple system atrophy. *J. Neurosci. Methods* **87**:111–115.

Braak H, Del Tredici K, Bratzke H, *et al.* (2002). Staging of the intracerebral inclusion body pathology associated with idiopathic Parkinson's disease (preclinical and clinical stages). [Review] [21 refs] *J. Neurol.* **249**(Suppl 3):III:1–5.

Braak H, Del Tredici K, Rub U, *et al.* (2003). Staging of brain pathology related to sporadic Parkinson's disease. *Neurobiol. Aging* **24**:197–211.

Burn DJ, Jaros E (2001). Multiple system atrophy: cellular and molecular pathology. [Review] *Mol. Pathol.* **54**:419–426.

Cairns NJ, Atkinson PF, Hanger DP, *et al.* (1997). Tau protein in the glial cytoplasmic inclusions of multiple system atrophy can be distinguished from abnormal tau in Alzheimer's disease. *Neurosci. Lett.* **230**:49–52.

Cannizzaro C, Tel BC, Rose S, *et al.* (2003). Increased neuropeptide Y mRNA expression in striatum in Parkinson's disease. *Brain Res. Mol. Brain Res.* **110**:169–176.

Choi W, Zibaee S, Jakes R, *et al.* (2004). Mutation E46K increases phospholipid binding and assembly into filaments of human alpha-synuclein. *FEBS Lett.* **576**:363–368.

Cilia R, Marotta G, Benti R, *et al.* (2005). Brain SPECT imaging in multiple system atrophy. *J. Neural Transmiss.* **112**:1635–1645.

Clarimon J, Johnson J, Djaldetti R, *et al.* (2005). Mutation of the Parkin gene in a Persian family: clinical progression over a 40-year period. *Mov. Dis.* **20**:887–890.

Conway KA, Harper JD, Lansbury PT (1998). Accelerated *in vitro* fibril formation by a mutant alpha-synuclein linked to early-onset Parkinson disease. *Nature Med.* **4**(11):1318–1320.

Colisimo C, Albanese A, Hughes AJ, *et al.* (1995). Some specific clinical features differentiate multiple system atrophy (striatonigral variety) from Parkinson's disease. *Arch. Neurol.* **54**:294–298.

Cousins DA, Burton EJ, Burn D, *et al.* (2003). Atrophy of the putamen in dementia with Lewy bodies but not Alzheimer's disease: an MRI study. *Neurology* **61**:1191–1195.

Critchley M (1929). Arteriosclerotic parkinsonism. *Brain* **52**:23–83.

Del Tredici K, Rub U, De Vos RA, *et al.* (2002). Where does parkinson disease pathology begin in the brain? *J. Neuropathol. Exp. Neurol.* **61**:413–426.

Dickson DW, Schmidt ML, Lee VM, *et al.* (1994). Immunoreactivity profile of hippocampal CA2/3 neurites in diffuse Lewy body disease. *Acta Neuropathol.* **87**:269–276.

Dickson DW, Lin W, Liu W-K, *et al.* (1999). Multiple system atrophy: a sporadic synucleinopathy. *Brain Pathol.* **9**:721–732.

Doubleday EK, Snowden JS, Varma AR, *et al.* (2002). Qualitative performance characteristics differentiate dementia with Lewy Bodies and Alzheimer's disease. *J. Neurol. Neurosurg. Psych.* **72**:602–607.

Duda JE, Giasson BI, Mabon ME, *et al.* (2002). Novel antibodies to synuclein show abundant striatal pathology in Lewy body diseases. *Ann. Neurology* **52**:205–210.

Eve DJ, Nisbet AP, Kingsbury AE, *et al.* (1997). Selective increase in somatostatin mRNA expression in human basal ganglia in Parkinson's disease. *Brain Res. Mol. Brain Res.* **50**:59–70.

Evidente VGH, Gwinn KA (1998). Neurological picture legend. Post-encephalitic parkinsonism. *J. Neurol. Neurosurg. Psych.* **64**:5.

Ferman TJ, Smith GE, Boeve BF, *et al.* (2004). DLB fluctuations: specific features that reliably differentiate DLB from AD and normal aging. *Neurology* **62**:181–187.

Forno LS (1969). Concentric hyalin intraneuronal inclusions of Lewy type in the brains of elderly persons (50 incidental cases): relationship to parkinsonism. *J. Am. Geriatr. Soc.* **17**:557–575.

Forno LS (1996). Neuropathology of Parkinson's disease. *J. Neuropathol. Exp. Neurol.* **55**:259–272.

Galvin JE (2003). Dementia with Lewy Bodies. *Arch. Neurol.* **60**:1332–1335.

Galvin JE, Giasson B, Hurtig HL, *et al.*(2000). Neurodegeneration with brain iron accumulation, type 1 is characterized by alpha-, beta-, and gamma-synuclein neuropathology. *Am. J. Pathol.* **157**:361–368.

Galvin JE, Lee SL, Perry A, *et al.* (2002). Familial dementia with Lewy bodies: clinicopathologic analysis of two kindreds. *Neurology* **59**:1079–1082.

Gasser T (2000). Autosomal-dominantly inherited forms of Parkinson's disease. [Review] [49 refs] *J. Neural Transmiss.* (Suppl.) **58**:31–40.

Gearing M, Lynn M, Mirra SS (1999). Neurofibrillary pathology in Alzheimer disease with Lewy bodies: two subgroups. *Archives of Neurology*, **56**:203–208.

Giasson BI, Mabon ME, Duda JE, *et al.* (2003). Tau and 14-3-3 in glial cytoplasmic inclusions of multiple system atrophy. *Acta Neuropathol.* **106**:243–250.

Gibb WR, Lees AJ (1987). The progression of idiopathic Parkinson's disease is not explained by age-related changes. Clinical and pathological comparisons with post-encephalitis parkinsonian syndrome. *Acta Neuropathol.* **73**:195–201.

Gibb WR. Lees AJ (1988). The relevance of the Lewy body to the pathogenesis of idiopathic Parkinson's disease. [Review] [41 refs] *J. Neurol. Neurosurg. Psych.* **51**:745–752.

Gilman S, Low PA, Quinn N, *et al.* (1999). Consensus statement on the diagnosis of multiple system atrophy. *J. Neurol. Sci.* **163**:94–98.

Gilman S, May SJ, Shults CW, *et al.*, and The North American Multiple System Atrophy Study Group (2005). The North American multiple system atrophy study group. *J. Neural Transmiss.* **112**:1687–1694.

Gomez-Tortosa E, Newell K, Irizarry MC, *et al.* (2000). Alpha-synuclein immunoreactivity in dementia with Lewy bodies: morphological staging and comparison with ubiquitin immunostaining. *Acta Neuropathol.* **99**:352–357.

Hansen L, Salmon D, Galasko D, *et al.* (1990). The Lewy-body variant of Alzheimer's disease: a clinical and pathologic entity. *Neurology* **40**:1–8.

Hansen LA, Samuel W (1997). Criteria for Alzheimer's disease and the nosology of dementia with Lewy bodies. *Neurology* **48**:126–132.

Hashimoto M, Kitagaki H, Imamura T, *et al.* (1998). Medial temporal and whole-brain atrophy in dementia with Lewy bodies: a volumetric MRI study. *Neurology* **51**:357–362.

Hayflick SJ, Westaway SK, Levinson B, *et al.* (2003). Genetic, clinical, and radiographic delineation of Hallervorden–Spatz syndrome. *N. Engl. J. Med.* **348**:33–40.

Hishikawa N, Hashizume Y, Yoshida M, *et al.* (2001). Widespread occurrence of argyrophilic glial inclusions in Parkinson's disease. *Neuropathol. Appl. Neurobiol.* **27**:362–372.

Hu XS, Okamura N, Arai H, *et al.* (2000). 18F-fluorodopa PET study of striatal dopamine uptake in the diagnosis of dementia with Lewy bodies. *Neurology* **55**:1575–1577.

Huang Y, Cheung L, Rowe D, *et al.* (2004). Genetic contributions to Parkinson's disease. [Review] [300 refs] *Brain Res. Brain Res. Rev.* **46**:44–70.

Hudson AJ, Rice GP (19990). Similarities of Guamanian ALS/PD to postencephalitic parkinsonism/ALS: possible viral cause. *Can. J. Neurol. Sci.* **17**:427–433.

Hughes AJ, Daniel S, Blankson S, *et al.* (1993a). A clinicopathologic study of 100 cases of Parkinson's disease. *Arch. Neurol.* **50**:140–148.

Hughes AJ, Daniel SE, Lees AJ (1993b). The clinical features of Parkinson's disease in 100 histologically proven cases. *Adv. Neurol.* **60**:595–599.

Inoue M, Yagashita S, Ryo M, *et al.* (1997). The distribution and dynamic density of oligodendroglial cytoplasmic inclusions (GCIs) in multiple system atrophy: A correlation between the densities of GCI and the degree of involvement of striatonigral and olivoponto-cerebellar systems. *Acta Neuropathol.* **93**:585–591.

Jellinger KA (1991). Pathology of Parkinson's disease other than the nigrostriatal pathway. *Mol. Chem. Neuropathol.* **14**:153–197.

Jellinger KA (2001). Influenza RNA not detected in archival brain tissues from acute encephalitis lethargica cases or in postencephalitic Parkinson cases. *J. Neuropathol. Exp. Neurol.* **60**:1121–1122.

Jellinger KA, Duda J (2003). Chapter 9: Other neurodegenerative disorders: neurodegeneration with brain iron accumulation, type 1 (Hallervorden–Spatz disease). In: *Neurodegeneration: The Molecular Pathology of Dementia and Movement Disorders.* DW Dickson (ed). ISN Neuropathol. Press, Basel, pp. 394–399.

Jellinger K, Mizuno Y (2003). Chapter 4. Synucleinopathies: Parkinson's disease. In: *Neurodegeneration: The Molecular Pathology of Dementia and Movement Disorders.* DW Dickson (ed). ISN Neuropathol. Press, Basel, pp. 159–187.

Kato S, Saito M, Hirano A, *et al.* (1999). Recent advances in research on neuropathological aspects of familial amyotrophic lateral sclerosis with superoxide dismutase 1 gene mutations: neuronal Lewy-like hyaline inclusions and astrocytic hyaline inclusions. *Histol. Histopathol.* **14**:973–989.

Kobayashi K, Miyazu K, Katsukawa K, *et al.* (1992). Cytoskeletal protein abnormalities in patients with olivopontocerebellar atrophy: an immunocytochemical and Gallyas silver impregnation study. *Neuropathol. Appl. Neurobiol.* **18**:237–249.

Kume A, Takahashi A, Hashizume Y (1991). Neuronal cell loss of the nigrostriatal system in multiple system atrophy. *J. Neurol. Sci.* **117**:33–40.

Lantos P, Quinn N (2003). Multiple system atrophy. In: *Neurodegeneration: The Molecular Pathology of Dementia and Movement Disorders.* DW Dickson (ed). ISN Neuropathol. Press, Basel, pp.203–214.

Lewy FH (1912). Paralysis agitans. I. Pathologische anatomie. In: *Handbuch der Neurologie*. M Lewandowsky, G Abelsdorff (eds). Springer, Berlin, pp. 920–933.

Lewy FH (1913). Zur pathologischen anatomie der paralysis agitans. *DZ Nervenheik* **50**:50–55.

Lobotesis K, Fenwick JD, Phipps A, *et al.* (2001). Occipital hypoperfusion on SPECT in dementia with Lewy bodies but not AD. *Neurology* **56**:643–649.

Lorberboym M, Djaldetti R, Melamed E, *et al.* (2004). 123I-FP-CIT SPECT imaging of dopamine transporters in patients with cerebrovascular disease and clinical diagnosis of vascular parkinsonism. *J. Nucl. Med.* **45**:1688–1693.

McKeith IG, Galasko D, Kosaka K, *et al.* (1996). Consensus guidelines for the clinical and pathologic diagnosis of dementia with Lewy bodies (DLB): Report of the consortium on DLB international workshop. *Neurology* **47**:1113–1124.

McKeith IG, Perry EK, Perry RH (1999). Report of the second dementia with Lewy body international workshop: diagnosis and treatment. Consortium on dementia with Lewy bodies. [Review] [34 refs] *Neurology* **53**:902–905.

McKeith IG, Ballard CG, Perry RH, *et al.* (2000). Prospective validation of Consensus criteria for the diagnosis of dementia with Lewy bodies. *Neurology* **54**:1050–1058.

McKeith I, Mintzer J, Aarsland D, *et al.* (2004). International Psychogeriatric Association Expert Meeting on DLB. Dementia with Lewy bodies. *Lancet Neurol.* **3**:19–28.

McKeith IG, Dickson DW, Lowe J, *et al.*, Consortium on DLB (2005). Diagnosis and management of dementia with Lewy bodies: third report of the DLB Consortium. *Neurology* **65**:1863–1872.

Middelkoop HAM, van der Flier WM, Burton EJ, *et al.* (2001). Dementia with Lewy bodies and AD are not associated with occipital lobe atrophy on MRI. *Neurology* **57**:2117–2120.

Miller GW, Erickson JD, Perez JT, *et al.* (1999). Immunochemical analysis of vesicular monoamine transporter (VMAT2) protein in Parkinson's disease. *Exp. Neurol.* **156**:138–148.

Mirra SS, Heyman A, McKeel D Jr, *et al.* (1991). The Consortium to Establish a Registry for Alzheimer's Disease (CERAD). Part II. Standardization of the neuropathologic assessment of Alzheimer's disease. *Neurology* **41**:479–486.

Morris HR (2005). Genetics of Parkinson's disease. [Review] [101 refs] *Ann. Med.* **37**(2):86–96.

Nisbet AP, Eve DJ, Kingsbury AE, *et al.* (1996). Glutamate decarboxylase-67 messenger RNA expression in normal human basal ganglia and in Parkinson's disease. *Neuroscience* **75**:389–406.

Noe E, Marder K, Bell KL, *et al.* (2003). Comparison of Dementia with Lewy bodies to Alzheimer's disease and Parkinson's disease with dementia. *Mov. Disord.* **19**(1):60–67.

Nurmi E, Ruottinen HM, Bergman J, *et al.* (2001). Rate of progression in Parkinson's disease: a 6-[18F]-fluoro-L-dopa PET study. *Mov. Disord.* **16**:608–615.

Ohara K, Takauchi S, Kokai M, *et al.* (1999). Familial dementia with Lewy bodies. *Clin. Neuropathol.* **5**:232–239.

Ozawa T, Paviour D, Quinn NP, *et al.* (2004). The spectrum of pathological involvement of the striatonigral and olivopontocerebellar systems in multiple system atrophy: clinicopathological correlations. *Brain* **127**(12):2657–2671.

Pakrasi S, O'Brien JT (2005). Emission tomography in dementia. [Review] [102 refs] *Nucl. Med. Comm.* **26**:189–196.

Paisan-Ruiz C, Lang AE, Kawarai T, *et al.* (2005). LRRK2 gene in Parkinson disease: mutation analysis and case control association study. *Neurology* **65**:696–700.

Pals P, Lincoln S, Manning J, *et al.* (2004). Alpha-synuclein promoter confers susceptibility to Parkinson's disease. *Ann. Neurol.* **56**:591–595.

Parkinson J (Sir James) (1817). 'An essay on the shaking palsy,' Whittingham and Rowland for Sherwood, Neely, and Jones, London.

Polymeropoulos MH, Lavedan C, Leroy E, *et al.* (1997). Mutation in the a-synuclein gene identified in families with Parkinson's disease. *Science* **276**:2045–2047.

Racette BA, Perry A, D-Avossa G, *et al.* (2001). Late-onset neurodegeneration with brain iron accumulation type 1: expanding the clinical spectrum. *Mov. Disord.* **16**:1148–1152.

Rampello L, Alvano A, Battaglia G, *et al.* (2005). Different clinical and evolutional patterns in late idiopathic and vascular parkinsonism. *J. Neurol.* **252**:1045–1049.

Ramsden DB, Parsons RB, Ho SL, *et al.* (2001). The aetiology of idiopathic Parkinson's disease. [Review] [183 refs] *Mol. Pathol.* **54**(6):369–380.

Rinne JO, Rummukainen J, Paljarvi L, *et al.* (1989). Dementia in Parkinson's disease is related to neuronal loss in the medial substantia nigra. *Ann. Neurol.* **26**:47–50.

Sakamoto M, Uchihara T, Nakamura A, *et al.* (2005). Progressive accumulation of ubiquitin and disappearance of alpha-synuclein epitope in multiple system atrophy-associated glial cytoplasmic inclusions: triple fluorescence study combined with Gallyas-Braak method. *Acta Neuropathol.* **110**:417–425.

Sandmann-Keil D, Braak H, Okochi M, *et al.* (1999). Alpha-synuclein immunoreactive Lewy bodies and Lewy neurites in Parkinson's disease are detectable by an advanced silver-staining technique. *Acta Neuropathol.* **98**:461–464.

Sibon I, Fenelon G, Quinn NP, *et al.* (2004). Vascular parkinsonism. [Review] [102 refs] *J. Neurol.* **251**:513–524.

Sibon I, Tison F (2004). Vascular parkinsonism. [Review] [53 refs] *Curr. Opin. Neurol.* **17**:49–54.

Snyder H, Wolozin B (2004). Pathological proteins in Parkinson's disease: focus on the proteasome. [Review] [179 refs] *J. Mol. Neurosci.* **24**:425–442.

Spargo E, Papp MI, Lantos PL (1996). Decrease in neuronal density in the cerebral cortex in multiple system atrophy. *Eur. J. Neurol.* **3**:450–456.

Thanvi B, Lo N, Robinson T (2005). Vascular parkinsonism: an important cause of parkinsonism in older people. [Review] [35 refs] *Age & Ageing* **34**:114–119. [Comment: Turnbull C (2005). *Age & Ageing* **34**:97–98.]

Thomas M, Hayflick SJ, Jankovic J (2004). Clinical heterogeneity of neurodegeneration with brain iron accumulation (Hallervorden–Spatz syndrome) and pantothenate kinase-associated neurodegeneration. *Mov. Disord.* **19**:36–42.

Tu PH, Galvin JE, Baba M, *et al.* (1998). Glial cytoplasmic inclusions in white matter oligodendrocytes of multiple system atrophy brains contain insoluble alpha-synuclein. *Ann. Neurol.* **44**:415–422.

Turnbull C (2005). Vascular parkinsonism: an important update. *Age & Ageing* **34**:97–98. [Comment on: Thanvi et al. (2005). *Age & Ageing* **34**:114–119.]

Uchihara T, Nakamura A, Mochizuki Y, *et al.* (2005). Silver stainings distinguish Lewy bodies and glial cytoplasmic inclusions: comparison between Gallyas–Braak and Campbell–Switzer methods. *Acta Neuropathol.* **110**:255–260.

Valente PM, Abou-Sleiman PM, Caputo V, *et al.* (2004). Hereditary early-onset Parkinson's disease caused by mutations in PINK1. *Science* **304**:1158–1160.

Vaughan JR, Farrer MJ, Wszolek ZK, *et al.* (1998). Sequencing of the alpha-synuclein gene in a large series of cases of familial Parkinson's disease fails to reveal any further mutations. The European Consortium on Genetic Susceptibility in Parkinson's Disease (GSPD). *Hum. Mol. Genet.* **7**:751–753.

Wakabayashi K, Yoshimoto M, Fukushima T, *et al.* (1999). Widespread occurrence of alpha synuclein/NACP-immunoreactive neuronal inclusions in juvenile and adult-onset Hallervorden–Spatz disease with Lewy bodies. *Neuropathol. Appl. Neurobiol.* **25**:363–368.

Wenning GK, Ben-Shlomo Y, Magalhaes M, *et al.* (1994). Clinical features and natural history of multiple system atrophy. An analysis of 100 patients. *Brain* **117**:835–845.

Wong KT, Allen IV, McQuaid S, *et al.* (1996). An immunohistochemical study of neurofibrillary tangle formation in postencephalitic parksinsonism. *Clin. Neuropathol.* **15**:22–25.

Yoshimura N, Yoshimura I, Asada M, *et al.* (1988). Juvenile Parkinson's disease with widespread Lewy bodies in the brain. *Acta Neuropathol.* **77**:213–218.

Zhou B, Westaway SK, Levinson B, *et al.* (2001). A novel pantothenate kinase gene (PANK2) is defective in Hallervorden–Spatz syndrome. *Nat. Genet.* **28**:345–349.

Zijlmans JC, Thijssen HO, Vogels OJ, *et al.* (1995). MRI in patients with suspected vascular parkinsonism. *Neurology* **45**:2183–2188.

Zijlmans JC, Daniel SE, Hughes AJ, *et al.* (2004). Clinicopathological investigation of vascular parkinsonism, including clinical criteria for diagnosis. *Mov. Disord.* **19**(6):630–640.

Chapter 8

The frontotemporal dementias

Introduction

A heterogeneous spectrum of disorders, collectively referred to as frontotemporal dementia (FTD), is associated with degeneration in the frontal and anterior temporal lobes. The clinical, neuroimaging, and pathologic presentation of each of these disorders and their relationship to the tau protein will be discussed briefly in this chapter.

The predominant pathologic involvement of the prefrontal cortex and anterior temporal lobes in these disorders is reflected by clinical syndromes characterized by various degrees of disturbed personality, behavior, and language (Neary *et al.*, 1998). While FTDs are the third most common form of neurodegenerative dementia behind Alzheimer's disease (AD) and dementia with Lewy bodies (DLB), accounting for perhaps 5–20% of all dementia cases

by various estimates, FTD is among the most common causes of early-onset dementia. FTD is rare in individuals over the age of 75 years and has a mean age at onset of 58 years (Ratnavalli *et al.*, 2002). In dementia patients with onset of dementia under 65 years, FTD accounts for perhaps 20% of neurodegenerative dementias. The usual duration of FTD is about 8–11 years and the clinical course is marked by faster rates of cognitive and functional decline compared to individuals with AD (Rascovsky *et al.*, 2005). Many individuals with FTD have a clear family history (Van Deerlin *et al.*, 2003).

To facilitate the identification and systematic study of this group of patients, several sets of research criteria have been proposed (*Table 8.1*) (Neary *et al.*, 1998; McKhann *et al.*,

Table 8.1 Frontotemporal lobar degenerations: clinical criteria

	Frontotemporal dementia	Progressive nonfluent aphasia	Semantic dementia
Core features	• Decline in social and personal conduct • Blunted emotions • Lack of insight	• Nonfluent speech with prominent anomia, agrammatism, and paraphasias	• Fluent speech lacking meaning • Prominent comprehension difficulties • Preserved drawing reproduction, single word repetition, ability to read aloud, and write to dictations
Supportive features	• Decline in personal hygiene • Dietary changes • Perseveration • Stereotyped behavior • Late mutism	• Stuttering • Alexia • Agraphia • Late behavioral changes	• Pressured speech • Loss of sympathy or empathy

(Neary *et al.*, 1998)

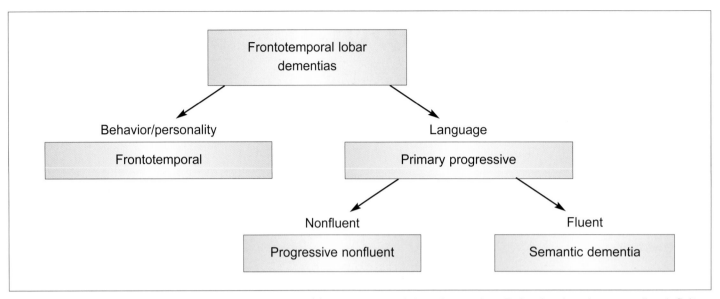

8.1 A diagrammatic depiction of the main subtypes of frontotemporal lobar dementias. Behavioral and personality deficits are related to frontotemporal pathology. The language deficit triad includes two subtypes of primary progressive aphasia: progressive nonfluent aphasia and fluent aphasia that is now referred to as semantic dementia.

2001). Broadly, these research criteria divide the clinical presentation of FTDs into behavioral and language syndromes. The language presentation of FTD is often referred to as primary progressive aphasia and, based on the presence of fluent or nonfluent speech output, can be further classified as progressive nonfluent aphasia and semantic dementia (**8.1**). The three syndromes tend to overlap and as each disease progresses, the clinical symptoms tend to converge, eventually resulting in mutism and behavioral disturbance. Similar features can occur with AD but are typically less pronounced and occur later in the course. FTD is often strikingly asymmetric, with variations in the extent and distribution of pathology. Additionally, there can be motor presentations. Some FTD patients develop a parkinsonian syndrome, which has been linked to mutations on chromosome 17, while others have associated motor neuron disease. The clinical heterogeneity makes diagnosis challenging and classifying the symptoms of FTD into discrete groups has been difficult, highlighting the need for a common set of assessment tools and diagnostic criteria to improve the identification and evaluation of individuals with language and behavioral decline.

While it is common for clinicians to refer to FTD as Pick's disease (PiD), PiD is a neuropathologic diagnosis that accounts for a minority of cases of FTD (15%). The original conception of PiD arose in the early 20th century from Arnold Pick's descriptions of focal atrophy on gross pathologic inspection of the brain from patients with personality changes and progressive aphasia (Pick, 1892). Alois Alzhiemer later described the intraneuronal inclusions that eventually became known as Pick bodies. The concept of PiD has expanded clinically and pathologically and the disorder has become known by multiple names including FTD, frontal lobe degeneration of the non-Alzheimer type, frontotemporal lobar degeneration, dementia lacking distinct histopathology (DLDH), primary progressive aphasia, and semantic dementia. The term Pick complex has been suggested as a unifying concept for these overlapping clinical disorders (Kertesz & Munoz, 1998).

Clinical features

Behavioral presentation

The clinical symptoms of FTD include early behavioral dysfunction with disinhibition, impulsivity, impaired judgment, and disturbed social comportment. Severe amnesia and visuospatial impairment are typically not present. In fact, many FTD patients are oriented and able to keep track of day-to-day affairs. Common features of the behavioral disturbance include inappropriate behavior such as swearing, off-color jokes, and loss of social tact. Patients are typically unconcerned about their appearance and hygiene. Some individuals develop repetitious or compulsive behavior. Dietary habits may change with the development of food fads in which only certain foods are eaten (often sweets). Patients can develop impulsiveness and distractibility. Individuals with FTD often have a dramatic loss of empathy along with a lack of insight into their personality changes and the impact these changes have on their family and friends.

Language presentation: primary progressive aphasia

The language presentation of FTD is characterized by a progressive change in language function in the setting of a relative preservation of other cognitive domains such as memory. The speech disturbance can involve fluent and nonfluent speech as a result of the anatomical distribution of the pathology. The left cerebral hemisphere is dominant for language. Wernicke's area is located in the left temporoparietal junction and mediates the sensory associations encoding word meaning. Broca's area is located in the inferior and middle gyri of the left frontal lobe, and is involved in generating articulatory sequences to transform thoughts into statements. These two centers are interconnected as part of the distributed language network and their differential involvement in the neurodegenerative process underlying FTD is responsible for the various speech disturbances associated with the disorder.

Progressive nonfluent aphasia

Progressive nonfluent aphasia (PNFA) is characterized by early loss of fluent speech and prominent anomia (**8.2**). The speech may have a halting quality due to frequent pauses for word-finding. Common features include circumlocutions in which articulation of thoughts is circuitous due to difficulty retrieving the concise words, and paraphasias in which incorrect words are substituted for the desired word. Speech

8.2 Structural MRI (MPRAGE) (top row) and PET images (bottom row) from a 72-year-old right handed woman with a 1-year history of progressive cognitive impairment primarily with difficulties in language. Her husband described her as having progressive difficulty with word-finding and 'difficulty structuring her sentences'. Her speech was nonfluent with frequent paraphasic errors. MRI revealed global atrophy slightly increased in the left temporal *vs.* right temporal lobe (arrowhead) as suggested by increased ventricular volume on the left. PET scanning revealed significant metabolic change in the left frontal lobes. The structural and imaging findings are consistent with a diagnosis of PNFA.

may be simplified through the use of generic words or rely on fillers such as 'thing' in place of the missing word. In some patients, the signs may be confined to the language areas for as many as 10 years. Eventually impairments emerge in other domains, although the language dysfunction remains the prominent symptom.

Semantic dementia

Semantic dementia (SD) is marked by early impairment in semantics (word meaning) resulting in empty, fluent speech and a loss of speech comprehension. Speech production may be effortless and without hesitancies but little meaningful information is conveyed. These subjects will have prominent comprehension problems (i.e. following commands), although impairment may not be immediately apparent in conversation because of the effortless speech. Because the language network prominently involved (Wernicke's area) abuts the visual association networks, semantic dementia may also be associated with complex visuoperceptual dysfunction such as prosopagnosia and visual object recognition.

Diagnosis

Clinical

The clinical diagnosis of FTD is made primarily based on the presence of behavioral symptoms leading to impairment in social or occupational function. Other potential medical causes must be ruled out such as cerebral mass lesions (tumor), cerebrovascular disease, Huntington disease, Parkinson's disease (PD), as well as systemic conditions that may cause dementia syndromes (hypothyroidism, human immunodeficiency virus). Three major anatomy-based clinical variants are currently recognized in the most general category of FTD: (1) a bifrontal subtype with slightly asymmetric, right frontotemporal region selective involvement, called frontotemporal dementia or the frontal variant of FTD (fvFTD); (2) a temporal predominant subtype called the temporal variant of FTD or SD; and (3) a left frontal predominant subtype, PNFA (Boxer & Miller, 2005).

Consensus clinical and pathologic definitions may facilitate diagnosis of this complex set of disorders (*Table 8.1*) (McKhann *et al.*, 2001). The demographics of 353 cases of FTD patients have recently been described (Johnson *et al.*, 2005). Onset age differed among the three

major clinical groups of FTD (57.5 years), semantic dementia (59.3 years), and progressive nonfluent dysphasia (PNFD) (63.0 years). Men predominated in the FTD (63.5%) and SD (66.7%) groups when compared to PNFA (39.1%).

Neuroimaging

Brain imaging should be obtained to rule out the presence of structural lesions and may reveal the presence of disproportionate atrophy in the frontal and temporal lobes (**8.3**). Additionally, functional imaging in the form of positron emission tomography (PET) or single photon emission computed tomography (SPECT) may reveal altered metabolic activity in the frontal and temporal lobes (**8.4**), the presence of which can be helpful in distinguishing the syndrome from AD which is associated with parietal lobe metabolic dysfunction. At times the degree of involvement structurally and functionally may be strikingly asymmetric.

MRI structural (T1-weighted) brain scans of persons with FTD reveal selective frontotemporal atrophy with disproportionately dilated frontal horns (Bocti *et al.*, 2006) (*Box 8.1*). Progressive hippocampal atrophy is a recognized feature of FTD (Laakso *et al.*, 2000). In contrast to AD, PET and functional MRI show predominant frontal attenuation of brain metabolic markers, whereas the commonest pattern observed in AD is superior parietotemporal hypometabolism and activation deficits (Buchert *et al.*, 2005; Zahn *et al.*, 2005).

Box 8.1 FTD patterns of atrophy: a new staging scheme

Patterns of brain atrophy in two coronal slices of 24 FTD cases staged from least (Stage 1) to most (Stage 4) severe that correlated with disease duration and clinical dementia severity

- Stage 1 – mild atrophy in orbital and medial superior frontal cortex and hippocampus
- Stage 2 – progression to involve other frontal regions, temporal cortices, and basal ganglia
- Stage 3 – involvement of all remaining tissue in the two coronal slices
- Stage 4 – very marked atrophy in all areas

(Mann & South, 1993; Broe *et al.*, 2003.)

8.3 Coronal and transverse MRI of a 73-year-old right-handed man with 3-year history of progressive memory impairment and behavioral changes. The MRI revealed significant global atrophy most prominent in the right frontal and temporal lobes. His symptoms began with cognitive decline (difficulty balancing checkbook, repeating questions) and were accompanied by significant behavioral changes. Early features included suspiciousness and paranoid delusions, socially inappropriate behavior, distractibility, and severe apathy. He was diagnosed with FTD. (Courtesy of Randy L Buckner, and the Washington University ADRC Neuroimaging Core Laboratory.)

8.4 PET imaging from a 64-year-old man with a 5-year history of progressive behavioral disturbance including reduced hygiene, hypersexuality, apathy, and a lack of insight into his problems. PET scanning revealed a dramatic decrease in metabolism of the frontal (arrows) and temporal (arrowhead) lobes with sparing of the parietal lobes (short arrow). Blue coloration in the PET images represents less metabolic activity while brighter (yellows and reds) coloration represents higher metabolic rates. The imaging findings are consistent with the clinical diagnosis of FTD.

Cerebrospinal fluid (CSF) protein biomarker analysis may be helpful in distinguishing FTD from other dementias. For example, tau phosphorylated at threonine 231 may provide excellent discrimination between AD and FTD (see *Box 8.2*).

Neuropsychology

Standard neuropsychological tests (Diehl *et al.*, 2005) and neuropsychiatric behavioral tests also may be used to distinguish FTD subtypes from other forms of dementia (Chow *et al.*, 2002) and depression (Elderkin-Thompson *et al.*, 2004). The differing test profiles between FTD and AD are portrayed in *Table 8.2* (Harciarek & Jodzio, 2005).

Box 8.2 CSF tau in the differential diagnosis of dementia

- Hyperphosphorylated tau (p-tau): Distinguishes AD from healthy controls
- Tau phosphorylated at serine181 (p-tau181): Enhances diagnosis of AD and DLB
- Tau phosphorylated at threonine 231 (p-tau231): Excellent discrimination between AD and FTD
- Total tau (t-tau): A general marker of neurodegeneration for evaluation in future population-based studies

(Hampel & Teipel, 2004)

Table 8.2 A simplified clinical-neuropsychological comparison of FTD and AD at the mild-moderate stage [1]

	FTD	AD
Clinical profile		
Prevalence among dementias (%)	~10	~70
Common presenting complaints	Personality/behavioral change	Forgetfulness
Neurologic/motor	Aberrant motor activity	Normal functioning
Neuropsychiatric	Apathy, loss of personal and interpersonal insight, impulsivity, disinhibition	Depression, anxiety, delusions
Course from diagnosis to death (years)	~8	~8–10
Progression	Gradual downward decline	Gradual downward decline
Neuropsychological profile		
Qualitative performance differences	Easily distracted, prone to impulsive and perseverative errors, poor self-monitoring	Forgetfulness for instructions, receptive language problems
Confusion/disorientation	+	+
Attention/concentration deficits	+++	++
Episodic memory deficits	++	++++
Language deficits	++	++
Executive dysfunction	++++	+++
Visuo-spatial deficits	–	+
ADL impairment	++	++

+: relative impairment in a given cognitive-functional domain when assessed at the mild to moderate stage of disease progression. Fewer + signs indicate less impaired functioning. -: relatively spared or normal functioning. FTD subtypes and related disorders involving the frontal and/or temporal lobes (e.g. PiD, PNFA, semantic aphasia) may present somewhat differently than is generally presented here. It is important to recognize that clinical presentations of these disorders will vary across individuals, especially when mixed dementia pathologies are present.

(Pasquier *et al.*, 1995; Binetti *et al.*, 2000; Smeding & de Koning, 2000; Siri *et al.*, 2001; Diehl & Kurz, 2002)

Neuropathology

Introduction and genetics

The FTDs are a non-AD family of dementing disorders based on the prototypic disorder PiD (*Table 8.3*). A common link between FTD entities is tau pathology (Brandt *et al.*, 2005), which may take several forms including several nonintuitive mechanisms of disease. Tau gene mutations on chromosome 17 may be found in approximately 25% of familial FTD cases (Goedert & Jakes, 2005). A comprehensive picture of FTD genetics is rapidly emerging that implicates not only tau gene mutations but also splice variants of tau (D'Souza & Schellenberg, 2005; Kar *et al.*, 2005) that alter tau isoform expression in a disease-specific manner (*Box 8.3*). Molecular, biochemical, and neuropathologic features have been used as a comprehensive scheme for classifying and differentiating the rapidly growing spectrum of FTD disorders (**8.5**).

Table 8.3 The major FTD disorder pathologic subtypes related to tau isoform expression

Disorder	Abnormal protein(s)	Typical clinical features	Typical pathologic features
Pick's disease	Tau (3R)	Dementia	• Anterior inferior 1/3 STG + prefrontal knife edge lobar atrophy pattern • Pick body • Pick cell
CBD	Tau (4R)	Dementia	• Asymmetric left > right cerebral atrophy (pre- and postcentral sulci) • Ballooned neuron • Astrocytic plaque • Glial and neuronal tau+ inclusions (WM) • WM massive tau+ neuritic pathology
PSP	Tau (4R)	Gaze palsy (specific), dementia	• Tangles with straight filaments in subcortex • Tufted astrocyte
FTDP-17	Tau (4R)	Bulimia, hyperphagia, behavioral abnormality, parkinsonism, dementia	• Frontal and temporal lobar atrophy, neuron loss, gliosis, nigral degeneration
DLDH	Soluble *vs.* insoluble tau abnormality	Dementia, FTD symptoms	• Frontotemporal atrophy, neuron loss, gliosis in the absence of tauopathy pathology
AGD	Tau (4R)	50% in nondemented, 50% demented, often with AD	• Limbic Gallyas and tau+ grains • Cortex layer 2 NFTs • WM coiled bodies and tau+ neurites • Amygdala ballooned neurons
FTD, familial	• Tau gene mutation on chromosome 17 • Tau protein misfolding • Tau posttranslational hyperphosphorylation	FTD personality disorder early, bulimia, psychosis, disinhibition, dysexecutive function deficits overlap sporadic FTD	• Tau DNA mutation • Increased or decreased soluble and insoluble brain tau burden • Tau splice variants cause abnormal isoform expression

Box 8.3 Tau-based biochemical classification of FTD

Twenty-one cases of FTD with tau and ubiquitin immunohistochemistry, tau isoform biochemistry, and Western blots[1]. Based on international diagnostic criteria by experts[2].

Neuropathologic criteria-based diagnosis:

- Classic PiD (n=7)
- CBD (n=5)
- PSP (n=2)
- DLDH (n=4)
  FTLD-MND/MNI (n=2)
- NFT dementia (n=1)

Insoluble tau distribution:

- 3R (n=5): 100% PiD
- 4R (n=7): 71% CBD, 29% PSP
- 3R/4R (n=3): 67% PiD + AD, 33% NFT dementia
- None (n=6): 67% DLDH, 33% FTLD-MND/MNI

[1]Mott *et al.*, 2005; [2]McKhann *et al.*, 2001

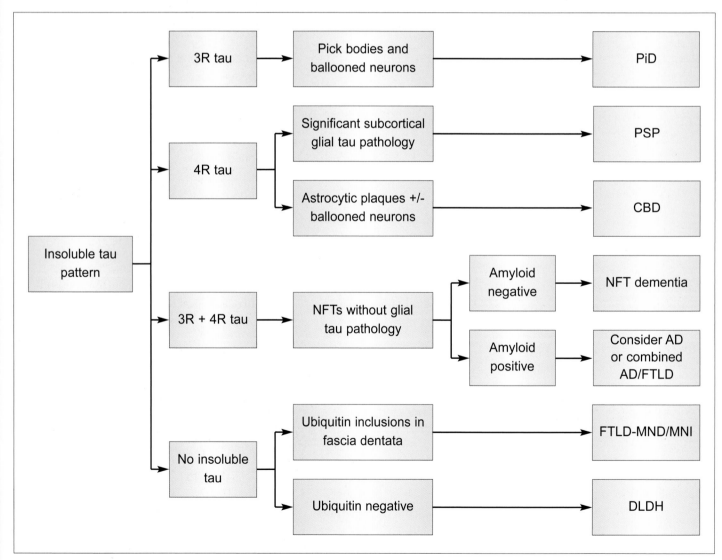

8.5 Diagnosis of dementia workflow.

Macroscopic and microscopic neuropathology

This family of neurodegenerative disorders has in common: (1) a molecular abnormality in the microtubule-associated protein tau (τ); (2) the pathologic burden falls disproportionately on the frontal and temporal lobes of the brain; and (3) the core pathologic features are lobar atrophy, cortical vacuolation with severe neuron loss, and astrocytic gliosis. Cerebral hemisphere atrophy may be symmetrical (**8.6**) or asymmetrical (**8.7**) in FTD. Superimposed on these core histologic features are various lesions, primarily types of cytoplasmic inclusions in neurons and glia and their processes, that morphologically define specific clinicopathologic disease entities classified within the broader FTD spectrum of neurologic diseases. *Table 8.3* lists the currently recognized major types of FTD. Broe *et al.* (2003) have proposed a four stage method for grading FTD pathologic severity.

8.6 This FTD brain shows relatively symmetrical hemispheral severe frontotemporal atrophy. Note the extreme thinning of the transverse corpus callosum and marked dilation of both frontal horns and the third ventricle. (Formalin-fixed autopsy specimen.)

8.7 Compared with the brain in **8.6**, this FTD coronal slice reveals striking asymmetrical atrophy with the left hemisphere (on the viewer's left) being significantly smaller than the right side. The corpus callosum is very thin and the anterior commissure demarcating the substantia innominata and basal forebrain is conspicuous. The caudate nuclei are thin and the left side is concave due to the expansion of the frontal horns (hydrocephalus *ex vacuo*), which is again asymmetric. Note the severe atrophy and disparity in volume of the left hemisphere white matter compared to the right. (Formalin-fixed autopsy specimen.)

Pick's disease

This is the prototypic disease among the frontotemporal dementing disorders. Understanding of the underlying biomolecular pathogenesis of PiD has increased dramatically in recent years (Dickson, 1998; Bergeron *et al.*, 2003; Uchihara *et al.*, 2005). Classical PiD atrophy pattern is pathognomonic (**8.8A**). The prefrontal cortex and anterior inferior third of the superior temporal gyrus (STG) are extremely shrunken with 'knife-edged' gyri. Affected brain has a tan-gray gelatinous appearance due to disappearance of white matter myelin secondary to severe cortical neuron loss and gliosis. The affected brain is firm and rubbery when cut. The rest of the brain is also atrophic; the degree depends on the total disease duration. However, the myelin in the parietal, occipital, and posterior two-thirds of STG and the remainder of the temporal lobe appear white and have a normal consistency. In the authors' experience, this pattern of atrophy is rare and is absolutely

predictive that Pick bodies and cells (ballooned neurons) will be present on microscopic examination. Cases of long-duration AD (i.e. >15 years total duration) may superficially resemble pure PiD (**8.8B**).

Coronal sections through the severely atrophic prefrontal and inferior temporal cortices in PiD reveal gray, rubbery tissue in which gray (GM) and white matter (WM) demarcation is blurred. The nonatrophic parieto-occipital cortices appear much more normal in the coronal plane, and the distinction between GM and WM is quite clear.

PiD cortex by H&E shows typical FTD neuron loss, gliosis, layer 2 microvacuoles (**8.9A, B**) and ballooned neurons called Pick cells (**8.9C**). Affected cerebral cortex and hippocampal CA1 in pure PiD contain Pick bodies that are intensely argyrophilic (Sevier-Munger silver, **8.10A, B**; Bielschowsky silver, **8.10D**) and tau positive (**8.10C**). Cortical and hippocampal Pick bodies differ from AD

8.8 A: The left lateral view of a classical Pick's disease brain reveals the pathognomonic cerebral atrophy pattern. The prefrontal lobe (facing left) is disproportionately shrunken as is the anterior and inferior portion of the temporal lobe. These areas when cut both had a tan color and felt rubbery when sectioned. In contrast, the posterior two-thirds of the temporal lobe and the parietal and occipital lobes (at right) had a normal gray-white matter junction with white myelin in the centrum semiovale even though these anatomic lobes shared in the atrophic pattern histologically. The cerebellum is relatively normal in size. (Formalin-fixed autopsy specimen.) **B**: Advanced cerebral atrophy in the left hemisphere of a brain from a patient with severe dementia and long-duration due to AD. Compare the more diffuse gyral atrophy that extends into the parietal and posterior temporal lobes to the classical PiD pattern in (**A**). The frontal lobe is at viewer's left and the occipital lobe and cerebellum are to the right. The latter appears normal. There is no selective atrophy of the anterior-inferior temporal lobe. Frontal lobe gyri display true 'knife-edge atrophy'. (Formalin-fixed autopsy specimen.)

8.9 A: PiD prefrontal lobe cortex shows the classic microscopic triad of FTD: microvacuolation centered in layer 2, severe neuron loss worse in the upper cortical layers, and diffuse transcortical gliosis. (H&E, ×10 objective.) **B**: Marked

reactive gliosis shown with GFAP immunostaining and a true blue substrate. (GFAP immunohistochemistry, ×10 objective.) **C**: A ballooned neuron 'Pick cell' with rounded soma and clearing of the central cytoplasm (asterisk) is shown in the frontal cortex. (H&E, ×40 objective.)

8.10 PiD frontal cortex (**A**) and hippocampal dentate fascia (**B**) neurons that contain numerous intensely argyrophilic Pick bodies with sharply defined edges and a dense homogenous substructure. Note that while most Pick bodies are circular, occasional ones in (**A**) are flame-shaped and extend into cell processes. (Sevier-Munger silver method, **A**: ×20 objective, **B**: ×10 objective.) (Courtesy of Dr Suzanne Mirra and the CERAD quality assurance program.) **C**: PiD cerebral cortex shows neurons with tau-positive Pick bodies and diffuse staining as

well as tau-positive neurites. (PHF-1 tau immunohistochemistry, ×10 objective.) **D**: Neuronal cytoplasmic Pick bodies (at center and 8 o'clock) also stain strongly with the modified Bielschowsky silver method. (mBT silver method [Washington University ADRC], ×40 objective.)

tangles in being: (1) more compact; (2) round or oval rather than flame-shaped; and (3) very discrete with sharply-defined borders. PiD and AD may co-occur; however, a-beta and argyrophilic senile plaques are not a feature of pure PiD. Mixed AD-PiD may show intermingling of neurofibrillary tangles (NFT) and Pick bodies such that high density regions for one lesion are low in the other and *vice versa* (McKeel *et al.*, 2000).

Corticobasal ganglionic degeneration

First described as primarily a motor neuron disease with initial asymmetric single limb involvement in the 1960s by Reibetz *et al.* (1967; 1968), CBD is now understood to be a more complex disorder with multiple clinical phenotypes, overexpression of 4-repeat tau isoforms, and frequent pathologic presentation as a mixed dementia (de Silva *et al.*,

2006). Tau, a 441 amino acid protein, has six isoforms in normal and AD brains, with a balanced ratio of 3 and 4 repeat isoforms (Dickson *et al.*, 2002) (**8.11**). Most cases of CBD are spontaneous, lack a defined tau or other gene mutation, and exhibit both clinical and pathologic heterogeneity as notable features in the extant literature (Schneider *et al.*, 1997; Boeve *et al.*, 1999; Doran *et al.*, 2003).

Macroscopic features of CBD brains (**8.12**) include asymmetric pre- and postparacentral sulcus widening that is more pronounced on the left compared to the right cerebral hemisphere (Boxer *et al.*, 2006). Cerebral hemisphere overall atrophy may also be more pronounced on the left side. AD brains usually feature symmetrical hemispheral atrophy. The substantia nigra is substantially depigmented and appears pale at autopsy.

1	441
1	412
1	383
1	410
1	381
1	352

8.11 Schematic diagram of the six human tau gene isoforms (352–441 amino acids) on chromosome 17 at q21. Alternative splicing of exon 2 (red), exon 3 (green), and exon 10 (yellow) results in the expression six tau protein isoforms. The microtubule-binding repeat portions of the molecule are shown as black bars. The top three isoforms have 4 repeats (4R-tau) and the three lower isoforms have only 3 repeats (3-R tau). (Adapted & Goedert, 2003.)

8.12 CBD brains may show asymmetrical atrophy with the left hemisphere being more affected than the right side as in this example. Characteristic atrophy patterns include selective widening of the paracentral region sulci. This change is seen to variable degrees in **A** and **B**. Note extreme 'limbic' temporal atrophy with extreme temporal horn dilation in the coronal section (**C**), with slightly more severe involvement of the left hemisphere. **D**: Striking pallor of the mid-brain SN that is common in CBD. (Formalin-fixed autopsy specimens.)

Microscopic features of CBD (**8.13A–D**) include focal ballooned neurons in premotor and cingulate cortex, widespread occurrence of tau immunoreactivity (antibodies AT8, PHF-1) in silver- (modified Bielschowsky and Gallyas methods) negative cortical neurons, presence of tau-positive astrocytic plaques (astrocytes with PHFtau-IR) in their distal processes (Feany & Dickson, 1995) predominately in affected neocortex, basophilic inclusions in residual nigral pigmented (dopaminergic) neurons that are Gallyas silver- and PHFtau-positive, and accumulation of white matter

8.13 A: Neuronal vacuolar degeneration (upper row and lower right panels) may occur in neurons with tau-positive (upper left), Gallyas silver (upper right), and modified Bielschowsky silver (lower right) staining in CBD. Occasional ballooned 'achromatic' neurons may be seen with the Gallyas silver method (lower left panel). The upper right and lower left Gallyas stained preparations also exhibit extensive neuritic pathology and staining of glia. (All panels ×40 objective.)
B: Astrocytic plaques are a highly characteristic pathologic feature of CBD neocortex and basal ganglia. The Gallyas method shows insoluble tau inclusions (lower left panel) in the distal processes of hypertrophic astrocytes. The Gallyas silver method (other three panels) is equally useful to demonstrate this lesion. So called tufted astrocytes, where the inclusions are centered in the cell body (soma), are more characteristic of PSP. Some argyrophilic inclusions in both CBD and PSP brains are difficult to classify (lower right panel). (Tau immunohistochemistry and Gallyas silver, ×40 objective.)
C: Extensive WM neuritic pathology that characterizes CBD. The Gallyas silver method (two left panels) and modified Bielschowsky silver method (mBT, upper right panel) also show WM 'coiled body' WM glial inclusions. The mBT method is less effective in demonstrating the neuritic component. (All panels ×20 objective.)
D: Basophilic inclusions (H&E stain, upper right) and severe neuronal pigmented (dopaminergic) neuron loss in the SN of the mid-brain are characteristic features of CBD. These nigral inclusions contain filamentous reticular (lower left), skein-like (lower right), and globoid inclusion material that stains with alz-50 (lower left) or PHF-1 tau (lower right) antibodies as well as with Gallyas silver (upper right). The latter structures resemble globoid Alzheimer-type NFTs. (All panels ×40 objective.)

oligodendroglial 'coiled bodies' (also Gallyas- and tau-positive) and copious Gallyas-/tau-positive WM dystrophic neurites. The tau lesions exhibit a superabundance of the 4-repeat (4R) form of the protein (Mott *et al.*, 2005). In all CBD cases the author has examined, tau-positive silver-negative inclusions occur in 20–40% of dentate fascia neurons. Also, the cerebellar dentate nucleus is always affected by Gallyas- and tau-positive inclusions of the large neurons, as well as by similarly staining coarse neurites confined to the gray matter of the nucleus.

Progressive supranuclear palsy (Steele–Richardson–Olszewski syndrome)

Clinical features of CBD and PSP are overlapping and distinction between the two disorders on clinical grounds alone may be difficult (Steele *et al.*, 1964; Morris *et al.*, 1999). At least two clinical phenotypes of PSP may be ascertained (*Box 8.4*). Tau- and silver-positive tangles that are 15 nm wide with straight filament morphology by electron microscopy accumulate in characteristic subcortical brain regions: subthalamic nucleus, globus pallidus, substantia nigra, and basis pontis. Senile plaques are not part of pure PSP; however, AD and PSP often co-exist (Gearing *et al.*, 1994). Tau pathology in cortical gray and white matter is generally less extensive than in CBD (Wakabayashi *et al.*, 2004).

Tufted astrocytes with dense tau-positive filaments in the glial cell body are a highly informative secondary feature of PSP brains (Iwasaki *et al.*, 2004; Josephs *et al.*, 2006). The cerebellar dentate nucleus may show 'grumose degeneration' in approximately 20–30% of PSP brains. This unusual lesion appears as perisomal coarse granular eosinophilic material that probably represents abnormal (possibly dissolving) synapses on dentate neuron cell bodies (somata). Figure **8.14** shows the microscopic appearance of PSP lesions.

Frontotemporal dementia with parkinsonism linked to chromosome 17

The tau gene is located on the long arm (21q) of chromosome 17 (Froelich *et al.*, 1999). The early cases were referred to by several names including 'frontal lobe dementia of non-AD type' (Brun, 1987), or simply as FTD. Parkinsonism became recognized as a prominent feature and was added later. FTDP-17, therefore, is derived from a generic term that applies to several disorders with a characteristic clinical profile (Foster *et al.*, 1997). Some

---

Box 8.4 Clinical phenotypes of PSP

103 cases of pathologically confirmed PSP formed two groups:

Richardson's syndrome (RS): 54% of total; 2/3 M
Shorter duration (5.9 years mean) and earlier death (72.1 years)
- Early onset of postural instability
- Falls
- Supranuclear vertical gaze palsy
- Cognitive dysfunction

PSP-parkinsonism (PSP-P): 33% of total;
M/F = 1:1
Longer duration (9.1 years) and later death (75.5 years)
- Asymmetric onset
- Tremor
- Moderate initial therapeutic response to levodopa
- Frequently confused with Parkinson's disease (PSP-P)

Unclassified: 14% – differed from first two types

(Williams *et al.*, 2005)

FTDP-17 cases have point or missense mutations of tau, of which more than thirty are now known (Hong *et al.*, 1998). Other cases belong to large pedigrees that have a characteristic haplotype but no known tau mutation. An example is the extensively studied hereditary dysphasic dementia with disinhibition (HDDD-2) pedigree (Lendon *et al.*, 1998; Johnson *et al.*, 2004).

Several neuropathologic phenotypes have been described in brains from affected FTDP-17 families: (1) a florid tauopathy with tau- and Gallyas silver-positive cortical GM and WM neurons, glial inclusions, and WM tau-positive neurites (Lendon *et al.*, 1998); (2) a phenotype that has only slight insoluble tau deposition by immunohistochemistry (see DLDH) (Lendon *et al.*, 1998); and (3) a different phenotype with ubiquinated hippocampal dentate fascia inclusions and inconspicuous tau pathology (Ghetti *et al.*, 2003; Shi *et al.*, 2005). Figure **8.15** shows extremely severe cerebral atrophy in a familial FTDP-17 case of unusually long duration.

8.14 PSP brains exhibit tangle-like tau immunoreactive structures in many subcortical regions of the cerebrum. This section of PSP pons shows a ballooned neuron (arrow), dense inclusions (arrowheads), and coarse granular cytoplasmic inclusions (short arrows). (PHF tau immunohistochemistry, ×40 objective.)

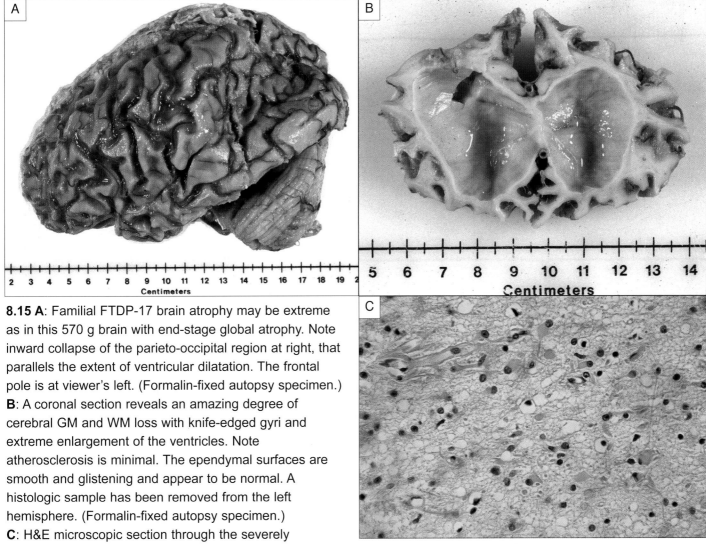

8.15 A: Familial FTDP-17 brain atrophy may be extreme as in this 570 g brain with end-stage global atrophy. Note inward collapse of the parieto-occipital region at right, that parallels the extent of ventricular dilatation. The frontal pole is at viewer's left. (Formalin-fixed autopsy specimen.)
B: A coronal section reveals an amazing degree of cerebral GM and WM loss with knife-edged gyri and extreme enlargement of the ventricles. Note atherosclerosis is minimal. The ependymal surfaces are smooth and glistening and appear to be normal. A histologic sample has been removed from the left hemisphere. (Formalin-fixed autopsy specimen.)
C: H&E microscopic section through the severely attenuated prefrontal cortex reveals almost total neuron loss, diffuse vacuolation in the neuropil attendant on neuron loss, and widespread occurrence of plump astrocytic gliosis. The elongated structure at upper left is a capillary. (H&E, ×40 objective.)

Dementia lacking distinctive histopathology

Brains from some individuals with the 'generic' FTD or FTDP-17 clinical phenotype are found at autopsy to lack distinctive pathologic features except for the core FTD features of severe frontotemporal neuron loss, gliosis, and superficial cortical microvacuolation (**8.16**) (Knopman *et al.*, 1990; Knopman, 1993). A series of elegant biochemical studies from the University of Pennsylvania Center for Neurodegeneration have shown that such brains have a marked abnormality in soluble and insoluble tau, both of which may be sharply decreased in brain homogenates (Zhukareva *et al.*, 2001). Recently, such cases have been identified to frequently harbor small ovoid ubiquinated but tau-negative inclusions in hippocampal dentate fascia neurons (**8.17**). The precise ubiquinated protein in such inclusions is not currently known. The dentate fascia ubiquitin-positive inclusions of FTD/DLDH are smaller than ones seen in CBD in 20–40% of dentate fascia neurons and lack tau immunoreactivity.

Argyrophilic grain disease

A relatively recently recognized disorder, AGD was described by Braak and Braak (1989) as a predominantly limbic disorder where the cardinal pathologic feature was comma or grape-like clusters of tau and Gallyas-silver 'grains' in neurons in the hippocampal CA1 region, the subiculum, the entorhinal allocortex, and the amygdala (**8.18A**, **C**). Three other defining features of AGD pathology include limbic cortex with superficial tau-positive tangles, 'coiled body' WM glial inclusions in limbic regions (**8.18D**), and ballooned neurons (that resemble Pick cells or premotor ballooned neuron [BN] in CBD) located in the amygdala (**8.18B**) (Togo & Dickson, 2002).

AGD is now recognized as a 4R tau disorder, as are CBD and PSP among the FTD disorders (see *Table 8.2*). It occurs in 20–25% of nondemented brains and as a sole lesion in some demented persons (Petersen *et al.*, 2006). AD is the most common dementia that is associated with AGD (Fujino *et al.*, 2005).

8.16 Dementia lacking distinctive histopathology neocortex from demented patients exhibits FTD core histopathologic features of severe neuron loss, microvacuolation of outer layers, and extensive gliosis in the absence of inclusions, SPs, NFTs, or other features of known dementias. Affected regions also appear grossly atrophic. (H&E, ×10 objective.)

8.17 Ubiquitin immunohistochemistry of DLDH brains, and FTD brains in general, reveals small cytoplasmic inclusions in upper layers of the neocortex (not shown) and in hippocampal dentate fascia neurons (arrows). The diagnostic inclusions are cytoplasmic, ovoid or kidney-shaped, small, and juxtanuclear in location as shown here. (Ubiquitin immunohistochemistry, ×40 objective.)

FTD tau mutation

Tau is a 441 amino acid protein with 13 exons, a hairpin loop structure where many mutations occur, multiple intronic (noncoding DNA) regions, and six normal isoforms in Western blots of normal human brains. Some tau mutations result in 'splicing in' exon 10 giving rise to 4R tau. Or, the mutation may cause deletion of exon 10 leading to overexpression of 3-repeat (3R) tau. Tau mRNA splicing abnormalities, or abnormal haplotypes involving chromosome 17 without a definite point (missense) mutation, are the pathologic basis for other cases of FTD. Figure **8.19** illustrates the appearance of anterior cingulate cortex stained by PHF-1 tau in the brain of an affected person carrying the R406W tau gene mutation (Reed *et al.*, 1997; Zhukareva *et al.*, 2003; Ostojic *et al.*, 2004; Zhukareva *et al.*, 2004).

8.18 AGD features four characteristic lesions: (1) 4R tau-positive and Gallyas silver-positive 'grains' (**A**: PHF-1 tau, **C**: Gallyas silver method with yellow arrow pointing to a grain); (2) ballooned neuron (arrow) in the amygdala (**B**: PHF-tau); (3) glial tau-positive (**D**: arrow) and Gallyas-positive coiled bodies; and (4) superficial layer temporal lobe NFTs (not shown). (**A**, **B**, and **D**: ×20, **C**: ×40 objectives.)

8.19 Anterior cingulate cerebral neocortex from a demented person carrying the autosomal dominant R406W tau gene mutation exhibits a dense mat of NTs and tau-positive neurons. The relatively poorly stained structure at lower right running diagonally across the field is the corpus callosum. (PHF-1 tau immunohistochemistry, ×20 objective.)

Neurofibrillary tangle dementia

The exact nosology of the emerging clinicopathologic entity NFT dementia is being defined (Jellinger & Bancher, 1998; Yamada, 2003). A subtype of AD with few or no senile plaques had been recognized in the early descriptive literature. Such cases and recent forensic descriptions of increased numbers of tangles in motor vehicle accident victims including elderly pedestrians (Gorrie *et al.*, 2006) may correspond to this newer presumptive nosologic entity of NFT dementia. In all cases, the pathology consists of dense NFTs of Alzheimer type that are largely confined to limbic regions. Amyloid senile plaques are rare or not present.

Mixed FTD

Several symptomatic types of FTD dementias may co-occur in the same individual. At autopsy the brains display diagnostic elements of both entities. Published recent reports include FTD and AGD (Ishihara *et al.*, 2005), amyotrophic lateral sclerosis (ALS) with PD and AGD (Liang *et al.*, 2005), FTD and motor neuron disease (Lipton *et al.*, 2004), and FTD with ALS and alpha-synuclein inclusion disease (Wilhelmsen *et al.*, 2004). PSP has been described in conjunction with AGD and AD (Liang *et al.*, 2005).

References

Bergeron C, Morris HR, Rossor M (2003). Chapter 3. Tauopathies: Pick's disease. In: *Neurodegeneration: The Molecular Pathology of Dementia and Movement Disorders*. DW Dickson (ed). ISN Neuropathology Press, Basel 2003, pp. 124–131.

Binetti G, Locascio JJ, Corkin S, *et al.* (2000). Differences between Pick disease and Alzheimer's disease in clinical appearance and rate of cognitive decline. *Arch. Neurol.* 57:225–232.

Bocti C, Rockel C, Roy P, *et al.* (2006). Topographical patterns of lobar atrophy in frontotemporal dementia and Alzheimer's disease. *Dementia Geriatr. Cogn. Disord.* 21:364–372.

Boeve BF, Maraganore DM, Parisi JE, *et al.* (1999). Pathologic heterogeneity in clinically diagnosed corticobasal degeneration. *Neurology* 53:795–800.

Boxer AL, Geschwind MD, Belfor N, *et al.* (2006). Patterns of brain atrophy that differentiate corticobasal degeneration syndrome from progressive supranuclear palsy. *Arch. Neurol.* 63:81-86

Boxer AL, Miller BL (2005). Clinical features of frontotemporal dementia. *Alz. Dis. Ass. Dis.* 19(Suppl. 1):S3–S6.

Braak H, Braak E (1989). Cortical and subcortical argyrophilic grains characterize a disease associated with adult onset dementia. *Neuropathol. Appl. Neurobiol.* 15:13–26.

Brandt R, Hundelt M, Shahani N (2005). Tau alteration and neuronal degeneration in tauopathies: mechanisms and models. (Review) (228 refs) *Biochim. Biophys. Acta* 1739:331–354.

Broe M, Hodges JR, Schofield E, *et al.* (2003). Staging disease severity in pathologically confirmed cases of frontotemporal dementia. *Neurology* 60:1005–1011.

Brun A (1987). Frontal lobe degeneration of non-Alzheimer type. I. Neuropathology. *Arch. Gerontol. Geriatr.* 6:193–208.

Buchert R, Wilke F, Chakrabarti B, *et al.* (2005). Adjusted scaling of FDG positron emission tomography images for statistical evaluation in patients with suspected Alzheimer's disease. *J. Neuroimag.* 15:348–355.

Chow TW, Miller BL, Boone K, *et al.* (2002). Frontotemporal dementia classification and neuropsychiatry. *Neurologist* 8:263–269.

de Silva R, Lashley T, Strand C, *et al.* (2006). An immunohistochemical study of cases of sporadic and inherited frontotemporal lobar degeneration using 3R- and 4R-specific tau monoclonal antibodies. *Acta Neuropathol.* (Berl) 111:329–340.

Dickson DW (1998). Pick's disease: a modern approach. *Brain Pathol.* 8:339–354.

Diehl J, Kurz A (2002). Frontotemporal dementia: patient characteristics, cognition, and behavior. *Int. J. Geriatr. Psych.* 17:914–918.

Dickson DW, Bergeron C, Chin SS, *et al.* (2002). Office of Rare Diseases neuropathologic criteria for corticobasal degeneration. *J. Neuropath. Exp. Neurol.* **61**:935–946.

Diehl J, Monsch AU, Aebi C, *et al.* (2005). Frontotemporal dementia, semantic dementia, and Alzheimer's disease: the contribution of standard neuropsychological tests to differential diagnosis. *J. Geriatr. Psych. Neurol.* **18**:39–44.

Doran M, du Plessis DG, Enevoldson TP, *et al.* (2003). Pathological heterogeneity of clinically diagnosed corticobasal degeneration. *J. Neurol. Sci.* **216**:127–134.

D'Souza I, Schellenberg GD (2005). Regulation of tau isoform expression and dementia. (Review) (117 refs) *Biochim. Biophys. Acta* **1739**:104–115.

Elderkin-Thompson V, Boone KB, Hwang S, *et al.* (2004). Neurocognitive profiles in elderly patients with frontotemporal degeneration or major depressive disorder. (Review) (136 refs) *J. Int. Neuropsychol. Soc.* **10**:753–771.

Feany MB, Dickson DW (1995). Widespread cytoskeletal pathology characterizes corticobasal degeneration. *Am. J. Pathol.* **146**:1388–1396.

Foster NL, Wilhelmsen K, Sima AA, *et al.* (1997). Frontotemporal dementia and parkinsonism linked to chromosome 17: a consensus conference. Conference participants. *Ann. Neurol.* **41**:706–715.

Froelich S, Houlden H, Rizzu P, *et al.* (1999). Construction of a detailed physical and transcript map of the FTDP-17 candidate region on chromosome 17q21. *Genomics* **60**:129–136.

Fujino Y, Wang DS, Thomas N, *et al.* (2005). Increased frequency of argyrophilic grain disease in Alzheimer disease with 4R tau-specific immunohistochemistry. *J. Neuropathol. Exp. Neurol.* **64**:209–214.

Gearing M, Olson DA, Watts RL, *et al.* (1994). Progressive supranuclear palsy: neuropathologic and clinical heterogeneity. *Neurology* **44**:1015–1024.

Ghetti B, Hutton ML, Wszolek ZK (2003). Frontotemporal dementia and parkinsonism linked to chromosome 17 associated with *Tau* gene mutations (FTDP-17). In: *Neurodegeneration: The Molecular Pathology of Dementia and Movement Disorders.* DW Dickson (ed). ISN Neuropathology Press, Basel, pp. 86–102.

Goedert M (2003). Introduction to the tauopathies. In: *Neurodegeneration: The Molecular Pathology of Dementia and Movement Disorders.* DW Dickson (ed). ISN Neuropathology Press, Basel, p. 82.

Goedert M, Jakes R (2005). Mutations causing neurodegenerative tauopathies. (Review) (139 refs) *Biochim. Biophys. Acta* **1739**:240–250.

Gorrie CA, Rodriguez M, Sachdev P, *et al.* (2006). Increased neurofibrillary tangles in the brains of older pedestrians killed in traffic accidents. *Dementia Geriatr. Cogn. Disord.* **22**:20–26.

Hampel H, Teipel SJ (2004). Total and phosphorylated tau proteins: evaluation as core biomarker candidates in frontotemporal dementia. (Review) (19 refs) *Dementia Geriatr. Cogn. Dis.* **17**(4):350–354.

Harciarek M, Jodzio K (2005). Neuropsychological differences between frontotemporal dementia and Alzheimer's disease: a review. *Neuropsychol. Rev.* **15**:131–145.

Hong M, Zhukareva V, Vogelsberg-Ragaglia V, *et al.* (1998). Mutation-specific functional impairments in distinct tau isoforms of hereditary FTDP-17. *Science* **282**:1914–1917.

Ishihara K, Araki S, Ihori N, *et al.* (2005). Argyrophilic grain disease presenting with frontotemporal dementia: a neuropsychological and pathological study of an autopsied case with presenile onset. *Neuropathology* **25**:165–170.

Iwasaki Y, Yoshida M, Hattori M, *et al.* (2004). Distribution of tuft-shaped astrocytes in the cerebral cortex in progressive supranuclear palsy. *Acta Neuropathol.* **108**:399–405.

Jellinger KA, Bancher C (1998). Senile dementia with tangles (tangle predominant form of senile dementia). *Brain Pathol.* **8**:367–376.

Johnson J, Ostojic J, Lannfelt L, *et al.* (2004). No evidence for tau duplications in frontal temporal dementia families showing genetic linkage to the tau locus in which tau mutations have not been found. *Neurosci. Lett.* **363**:99–101.

Johnson JK, Diehl J, Mendez MF, *et al.* (2005). Frontotemporal lobar degeneration: demographic characteristics of 353 patients. *Arch. Neurol.* **62**:925–930.

Josephs KA, Mandrekar JN, Dickson DW (2006). The relationship between histopathological features of progressive supranuclear palsy and disease duration. *Parkinsonism Rel. Dis.* **12**:109–112.

Kar A, Kuo D, He R, *et al.* (2005). Tau alternative splicing and frontotemporal dementia. *Alz. Dis. Assoc. Disord.* **19**:S29–S36.

Kertesz A, Munoz D (1998). Pick's disease, frontotemporal dementia, and Pick complex. *Arch. Neurol.* 55:302–304.

Knopman D, Mastri A, Frey W, *et al.* (1990). Dementia lacking distinctive histologic features: a common non-Alzheimer degenerative dementia. *Neurology* 40:251–256.

Knopman DS (1993). Overview of dementia lacking distinctive histology: pathological designation of a progressive dementia. *Dementia* 4:132–136.

Laakso MP, Frisoni GB, Kononen M, *et al.* (2000). Hippocampus and entorhinal cortex in frontotemporal dementia and Alzheimer's disease: a morphometric MRI study. *Biol. Psych.* 47:1056–1063.

Lendon CL, Lynch T, Norton J, *et al.* (1998). Linkage to chromosome 17q23 in hereditary dysphasic dementia, a frontotemporal dementia. *Neurology* 50:1546–1555.

Liang TW, Forman MS, Duda JE, *et al.* (2005). Multiple pathologies in a patient with a progressive neurodegenerative syndrome. *J. Neurol. Neurosurg. Psych.* 76:252–255.

Lipton AM, White CL 3rd, Bigio EH (2004). Frontotemporal lobar degeneration with motor neuron disease-type inclusions predominates in 76 cases of frontotemporal degeneration. *Acta Neuropathol.* 108:379–385.

Mann DMA, South PW (1993). The topographic distribution of brain atrophy in frontotemporal dementia. *Acta Neuropathol.* 85:334–340.

McKeel DW Jr (2000). The Alzheimer-Pick spectrum: mixed cases have 'mosaic' regions containing Pick bodies and PHFtau immunoreactive tangles. Abstract 155 accepted by the World Congress of Neuropathology, Birmingham, UK.

McKhann GM, Albert MS, Grossman M, *et al.* (2001). Clinical and pathological diagnosis of frontotemporal dementia: report of the Work Group on Frontotemporal Dementia and Pick's Disease. *Arch. Neurol.* 58:1803–1809.

Morris HR, Wood NW, Lees AJ (1999). Review: classic diseases revisited. Progressive supranuclear palsy (Steele–Richardson–Olszewski disease). *Postgrad. Med. J.* 75:579–584.

Mott RT, Dickson DW, Trojanowski JQ, *et al.* (2005). Neuropathologic, biochemical, and molecular characterization of the frontotemporal dementias. *J. Neuropathol. Exp. Neurol.* 64:420–428.

Neary D, Snowden JS, Gustafson L, *et al.* (1998). Frontotemporal lobar degeneration: a consensus on clinical diagnostic criteria. *Neurology* 51:1546–1554.

Ostojic J, Elfgren C, Passant U, *et al.* (2004). The tau R406W mutation causes progressive presenile dementia with bitemporal atrophy. *Dementia Geriatr. Cogn. Disord.* 17:298–301.

Pasquier F, Lebert F, Grymnprez L, *et al.* (1995). Verbal fluency in dementia of frontal lobe type and dementia of Alzheimer type. *J. Neurol. Neurosurg. Psych.* 58:81–84.

Petersen RC, Parisi JE, Dickson DW, *et al.* (2006). Neuropathologic features of amnestic mild cognitive impairment. *Arch. Neurol.* 63:665–672.

Pick A (1892). Uber die beziehungen der senilen hirnatrophie zur aphasie. *Praflw. Ated. Wochenschr.* 17:165–167.

Ratnavalli E, Brayne C, Dawson K, *et al.* (2002). The prevalence of frontotemporal dementia. *Neurology* 58:1615–1621.

Rascovsky K, Salmon DP, Lipton AM, *et al.* (2005). Rate of progression differs in frontotemporal dementia and Alzheimer disease. *Neurology* 65:397–403.

Rebeiz JJ, Kolodny EH, Richardson EP Jr (1967). Corticodentatonigral degeneration with neuronal achromasia: a progressive disorder of late adult life. *Trans. Am. Neurol. Assoc.* 92:23–26.

Rebeiz JJ, Kolodny EH, Richardson EP Jr (1968). Corticodentatonigral degeneration with neuronal achromasia. *Arch. Neurol.* 18:20–33.

Reed LA, Grabowski TJ, Schmidt ML, *et al.* (1997). Autosomal dominant dementia with widespread neurofibrillary tangles. *Ann. Neurol.* 42:564–572.

Schneider JA, Watts RL, Gearing M, *et al.* (1997). Corticobasal degeneration: neuropathologic and clinical heterogeneity. *Neurology* 48:959–969.

Shi J, Shaw CL, Du Plessis D, *et al.* (2005). Histopathological changes underlying frontotemporal lobar degeneration with clinicopathological correlation. *Acta Neuropathol.* (Berl) 110:501–512.

Siri S, Benaglio I, Frigerio A, *et al.* (2001). A brief neuropsychological assessment for the differential diagnosis between frontotemporal dementia and Alzheimer's disease. *Eur. J. Neurol.* 8:125–132.

Smeding HMM, de Koning I (2000). Frontotemporal dementia and neuropsychology: the value of missing values. *J. Neurol. Neurosurg. Psych.* 68:726–730.

Steele J, Richardson JC, Olszewski J (1964). Progressive supranuclear palsy. A heterogeneous system degeneration involving brainstem, basal ganglia, and cerebellum with vertical gaze and pseudobulbar palsy, nuchal dystonia, and dementia. *Arch. Neurol.* **10**:333–359.

Togo T, Dickson DW (2002). Ballooned neurons in progressive supranuclear palsy are usually due to concurrent argyrophilic grain disease. *Acta Neuropathol.* **104**:53–56.

Uchihara T, Tsuchiya K, Nakamura A, *et al.* (2005). Silver staining profiles distinguish Pick bodies from neurofibrillary tangles of Alzheimer type: comparison between Gallyas and Campbell-Switzer methods. *Acta Neuropathol.* **109**:483–489.

Van Deerlin VM, Gill LH, Farmer JM, *et al.* (2003). Familial frontotemporal dementia: from gene discovery to clinical molecular diagnostics. (Review) (74 refs) *Clin. Chem.* **49**:1717–1725.

Wakabayashi K, Takahashi H (2004). Pathological heterogeneity in progressive supranuclear palsy and corticobasal degeneration. (Review) (63 refs) *Neuropathology* **24**:79–86.

Wilhelmsen KC, Forman MS, Rosen HJ, *et al.* (2004). 17q-linked frontotemporal dementia-amyotrophic lateral sclerosis without tau mutations with tau and alpha-synuclein inclusions. *Arch. Neurol.* **61**:398–406.

Williams DR, de Silva R, Paviour DC, *et al.* (2005). Characteristics of two distinct clinical phenotypes in pathologically proven progressive supranuclear palsy: Richardson's syndrome and PSP-parkinsonism. *Brain* **128**(Pt 6):1247–1258. (Comment in: *Brain* 2005;**128**(Pt 6):1235–1236.)

Yamada, M (2003). Senile dementia of the neurofibrillary tangle type (tangle-only dementia): neuropathological criteria and clinical guidelines for diagnosis. *Neuropathology* **23**:311–317.

Zahn R, Buechert M, Overmans J, *et al.* (2005). Mapping of temporal and parietal cortex in progressive nonfluent aphasia and Alzheimer's disease using chemical shift imaging, voxel-based morphometry, and positron emission tomography. *Psych. Res.* **140**:115–131.

Zhukareva V, Sundarraj S, Mann D, *et al.* (2003). Selective reduction of soluble tau proteins in sporadic and familial frontotemporal dementias: an international follow-up study. *Acta Neuropathol.* (Berl) **105**:469–476.

Zhukareva V, Trojanowski JQ, Lee VM (2004). Assessment of pathological tau proteins in frontotemporal dementias: qualitative and quantitative approaches. *Am. J. Geriatr. Psych.* **12**:136–145.

Zhukareva V, Vogelsberg-Ragaglia V, Van Deerlin VM, *et al.* (2001). Loss of brain tau defines novel sporadic and familial tauopathies with frontotemporal dementia. *Ann. Neurol.* **49**:165–175.

Chapter 9

Neuropathology of miscellaneous dementing disorders

Introduction

Miscellaneous nonAlzheimer's disease (nonAD) neurodegenerative and dementing disorders increasingly must be considered in the differential diagnosis of the numerically most common forms of adult dementia: AD (beta amyloidoses), Lewy body disorders (alpha-synucleinopathies), frontotemporal dementia (FTD) (tauopathies, ubiquitinopathies), and vascular disorders (*Table 9.1*). In aggregate, this group of miscellaneous diseases may account for 10–15% of total adult dementia cases. The list is not exhaustive and these less common disorders are reviewed to emphasize the wide range of pathology that can cause dementia in adults.

Hippocampal sclerosis (HS)

A few percent of elderly brains show profound CA1 pyramidal neuron loss (80–90%) and gliosis as a primary histopathologic lesion (Dickson *et al.*, 1994; Corey-Bloom *et al.*, 1997; Ala *et al.*, 2000). The prevalence of hippocampal sclerosis (HS) was 13% of 382 dementia autopsies in a series from the State of Florida Brain Bank (Barker *et al.*, 2002). AD co-occurred with HS in 66% of the cases. Elderly HS pathology resembles HS seen by magnetic resonance imaging (MRI) during life and by pathologists in temporal lobe resection specimens from younger patients with intractable temporal lobe epilepsy. Epileptic HS is usually a unilateral disorder that can be lateralized

Table 9.1 Miscellaneous dementing disorders of adults

Dementing disorder	Abnormal protein
HS	None known (apoptosis cascade)?
Nucleotide repeat disorders: HD	Huntingtin gene mutation with increased 'CAG' repeats
Kuf's disease (ceroid lipofuscinosis)	Ceroid lipids NCL 1–9 gene mutation
Prion diseases (CJD, vCJD, FFI, GSS, kuru, BSE)	PrP_{sc} (sc = scrapie form)
Neurofilament inclusion body disease	Neurofilament subunits
ALS	aSYN, ubiquitin
Rare causes of acute dementia	Environmental toxins interacting with cellular metabolic and structural proteins
Causes of reversible dementia	Hypothyroidism, vitamin B_{12} deficiency, NPH
Multiple sclerosis: cognitive impairment	Not known

References for each dementing disorder are listed on page 182
NPH: normal pressure hydrocephalus

accurately by MRI and by electrophysiologic techniques (Fish & Spencer, 1995; Mintzer *et al.*, 2004). HS of the elderly is most often a bilateral medial temporal lobe and limbic lesion. The exact etiologic cause of either type of HS is not precisely known. In both conditions, however, excitotoxic glutamate-mediated or ischemic factors or both may play important roles.

Patients with cognitive impairment due mainly to HS, when they are followed longitudinally, may show slowly progressive memory impairment as the major clinical feature. HS pathology is seen in some cases of mild cognitive impairment (MCI) (Petersen *et al.*, 2006). Global dementing symptoms then may appear if HS co-occurs with AD. MRI of HS of the elderly often fails to show the lesion resulting in an erroneous diagnosis of MCI or incipient or mild AD. Thus, HS of the elderly is rarely diagnosed antemortem and is usually first detected at autopsy. Such HS cases may masquerade as AD in clinical drug trials and account for some of the commonly observed drug response heterogeneity among participants. AD nonresponders to anticholinergics, for example, may actually have HS which is not known to affect the cholinergic neurotransmitter system.

Recently, reports have suggested that most cases of HS may be examples of FTD motor neuron disease subtype (Hatanpaa *et al.*, 2004). Decreased grooming and inappropriate behavior were more common in HS and FTD than in AD. This assertion also was based on the finding that 61% of 18 HS cases studied harbored ubiquitin-positive inclusions in hippocampal dentate fascia (DF) neurons (Blass *et al.*, 2003). In the author's experience, HS cases usually do not have the core histopathologic features of FTD. That is, marked frontotemporal atrophy with severe prefrontal neuron loss, microvacuolation, and secondary gliosis are usually absent in nonAD HS brains. The full clinical and nosologic significance of DF ubiquinated inclusions remains to be clarified. This topic is also covered in Chapter 8 on FTD disorders.

Microscopic features of primary HS of the elderly (**9.1**) must be distinguished from the devastated hippocampal CA1 pathology in advanced long-duration AD. Brains with severe AD hippocampal pathology have extensive tangle formation. Many intraneuronal tangles have converted to the extracellular (ghost, tombstone) form that stain weakly with silver and H&E. Advanced AD pathology can thus mimic primary HS which lacks significant numbers of any type of neurofibrillary tangles (NFTs). One must remember, however, that a few hippocampal CA1 NFTs are an almost universal finding after age 60 years, so a few tangles might be expected even in primary HS.

9.1 A: Hippocampal area CA1 in primary HS on routine H&E staining shows almost total loss of recognizable pyramidal neurons. The field is instead dominated by proliferating astrocytes with star-shaped bright red processes (reactive gliosis). Special stains for Alzheimer SPs and NFTs are negative. **B**: A view of the subiculum shows marked atrophy of the gray matter (center third) marked by severe neuron loss and gliosis, bordered by normal appearing white matter occupying the upper and lower thirds of the field. (H&E, ×10 objective.)

Huntington's disease

Huntington's disease (HD) is a familial neurodegenerative disorder. The clinical picture is dominated by choreiform movement disorders and later by the advent of dementia (Andrews *et al.*, 1999). Gene expression causes progressive caudate nucleus atrophy (**9.2A**) (Aylward *et al.*, 2000) and hierarchical dorsal to ventral loss of caudate neurons (**9.2B**) (Vonsattel *et al.*, 1985; Hedreen *et al.*, 1991; Sotrel *et al.*, 1991; Heinsen *et al.*, 1994). Inheritance is autosomal dominant, high penetrance, with onset in the early 40s. In 1993 the causative gene IT 15, which is located on the short arm of chromosome 4 at 4p16.3 and encodes the protein *huntingtin* (htt), was isolated by the Huntington's Disease Collaborative group (1993). The huntingtin protein normally has a large number of CAG repeats at the N-terminus. This region of the molecule is expanded beyond 35 to varying degrees in affected HD subjects. In HD huntingtin protein aggregates form ubiquinated intranuclear inclusions (Sapp *et al.*, 1997). The molecular mechanisms underlying variability in the number of CAG repeats in different HD carriers and how the genotype determines the clinical phenotype are currently under active investigation in many centers (Persichetti *et al.*, 1994; Xuereb *et al.*, 1996).

Kuf's disease (neuronal ceroid lipofuscinosis [NCL])

Juvenile and adult forms of Kuf's disease result from excessive neuronal (and possibly glial) cytoplasmic storage of ceroid lipopigment (Mole *et al.*, 2005). The disease is sometimes called 'ceroid lipofuscinosis'. Most adult Kuf's cases are sporadic, but affected families with autosomal dominant inheritance have been reported (Josephson *et al.*, 2001).

Children with NCL suffer from visual failure, seizures, progressive physical and mental decline, and premature death, features associated with the loss of cortical neurons and accumulation therein of autofluorescent periodic acid-Schiff (PAS)-positive pigment resembling the aging pigment lipofuscin. The adult form of NCL, Kuf's disease, is far less common. Seven genes have been identified that cause human NCL (*CLN1*, *CLN2*, *CLN3*, *CLN5*, *CLN6*, *CLN8*, *CLN9*-deficit), and approximately 150 mutations have been described (all mutations are described in the NCL Mutation Database (http://www.uc.ac.uk/ncl) (*Box 9.1*). Clinically, two types of adult NCL are recognized, one with tonic–clonic seizures, the other with dementia (Josephson *et al.*, 2001). Rare familial cases exhibit early onset seizures, dementia, and motor abnormalities.

9.2 A: Hemibrain coronal slices from a normal age-matched control (left) and from an advanced stage HD (right). The main finding in HD is marked atrophy of the caudate nucleus. Note the caudate head is markedly flattened on the right compared to the normal convex curvature of the caudate on the left as it impinges into the ventricle. The angle of the frontal horn of the HD brain at right is also more rounded. (Formalin fixed autopsy specimen.) (Courtesy of Dr Robert E Schmidt.) **B**: Microscopically the caudate nucleus of an advanced HD person shows severe neuron loss and reactive astrocytic gliosis. Demarcation of the striosomes is blurred. The black arrow points to a probable residual neuron and the yellow arrow to a reactive astrocyte. Occasional microglia with rod-shaped nuclei and oligodendrocyte nuclei are scattered throughout the field. (H&E, ×40 objective.) (Courtesy of Dr Robert E Schmidt.)

Box 9.1 Neuronal ceroid lipofuscinosis[1] subtypes
- CLN1: Infantile (palmitoyl protein thioesterase deficiency [gene at the 1p32 locus])[2]
- CLN2: Late infantile mutations (pepstatin resistant proteinase deficiency (gen at the 11p15.5 locus)[3]
- CLN3: Juvenile (Batten's disease), 1.02 kb deletion on the CLN3 gene, CLN3 protein (specific gene [locus 16p11.2-12.3])[4]
- CLN5: Finnish variant of human late infantile NCL (13q21 locus)
- CLN6: Turkish variant late infantile NCL (15q21-23) (vLINCL)[5]
- CLN7: 'True' late infantile Turkish NCL[5]
- CLN8: Finland 1st case, all homozygous for a p.Arg24Gly mutation in CLN8; Turkish variant late infantile NCL (vLINCL)[6]
- CLN9-deficient[7]

[1]Seehafer & Pearce, 2006; [2]Bonsignore *et al.*, 2006; [3]Awano *et al.*, 2006; [4]Collins *et al.*, 2006; [5]Siintola *et al.*, 2005; [6]Cannelli *et al.*, 2006; [7]Schulz *et al.*, 2006

At autopsy the brain is grossly atrophic, the degree depends on the total duration of the disease. Microscopic examination using PAS or thioflavine S reveals grotesquely swollen and rounded ('ballooned') neurons throughout the cerebral cortex, cerebellum, subcortical nuclei, and the brainstem nuclei. There is no inflammatory reaction and glial reaction in the form of gliosis is mild or absent.

Examples of sporadic and familial Kuf's cases from the Washington University neuropathology registry are shown in Figure **9.3**.

Electron microscopy reveals the presence of curvilinear inclusions, fingerprint profiles, and granular osmiophilic deposits in neurons, lymphocytes, and conjunctival cells.

9.3 A: Adult form of NCL. The soma of cortical neurons (arrows) in the temporal lobe and elsewhere throughout this brain are enlarged and show a rounded contour due to excess stored lipopigment. **B:** Cortical neurons from a familial case of NCL have been stained with PAS and reveal stored lipopigment as coarse cytoplasmic granules that are larger than typical lipofuscin. Reactive gliosis or inflammation are not seen. (**A:** H&E, ×40 objective; **B:** PAS, ×40 objective.)

Prion diseases

The extent of prion-associated human diseases continues to expand as basic prion molecular and cellular pathobiology unfolds (Safar *et al.*, 2005; Priola & Vorberg, 2006). Creutzfeldt-Jakob Disease (CJD), the prototypic disease, has long been recognized as a rapidly fatal (95% less than 1 year from onset of initial symptoms until death) illness affecting persons in their 50s and 60s. Over 90% of CJD cases are sporadic and the rest are inherited (the gene or genes involved are not known) (Gambetti *et al.*, 2003). Carleton Gadjusek won the Nobel Prize in Medicine in 1976 for his pioneering work in elucidating the transmissible nature of this mysterious disorder (1976). Stanley Prusiner earned the same prize in 1997 for proving that prions are self-replicating infectious agents that are not viral or virus derived (1997).

We now know that the transmissible spongiform encephalopathies (TSE) are an important subset of dementing human diseases, the prionoses, that are all caused by various forms of prion agents (Chakraborty *et al.*, 2005). Besides the central nervous system and peripheral tissues and blood, PrP antigen also can be demonstrated immunohistochemically in the peripheral nervous system in ganglia (including autonomic) and in the dorsal horns of the spinal cord and the medullary sensory nuclei (Ishida *et al.*, 2005; Lee *et al.*, 2005). Because of the advent of variant forms of CJD, and the fact that these disorders are invariably and rapidly fatal, the NIH supports a United States National Prion Pathology Surveillance Center under Dr Pierluigi Gambetti's direction in the Department of Pathology at Case Western Reserve medical center in Cleveland, Ohio (website http://www.cjdsurveillance.com). Similar registries exist in Europe, in Australia (Klug *et al.*, 2005), and elsewhere.

Sporadic CJD

Clinically, sporadic CJD (sCJD) patients have corticospinal tract signs, develop myoclonus, have a unique spike pattern on electroencephalography (EEG), develop a high percentage (~95%) of the 14-3-3 protein in CSF, and terminally become demented, mute, and die (Van Everbroeck *et al.*, 2000). A 'Heidenhain variant' of sCJD that selectively affects vision is also recognized (Cooper *et al.*, 2005).

The neuropsychological profile of patients with classical sCJD differs markedly from that of AD patients (*Table 9.2*).

The core pathologic features of sCJD include severe brain atrophy and a constellation of lesions termed 'spongiform encephalopathy', namely, transcortical neuronal vacuolation, neuron loss, and astrocytic gliosis (Budka *et al.*, 2003). White matter and hippocampus may be severely affected. Some cases show milder cortical spongiform encephalopathy necessitating use of biomolecular techniques to base the diagnosis on particular known genotypes codon 129 and PrP molecular isoforms 1a (~21 kDa), 2a (sCJD, ~19 kDa), and 2b (vCJD) that may be analyzed by Western Blot or real-time polymerase chain reaction (RT-PCR), and immunohistochemical delineation of the pathologic agent using specific anti PrP-scrapie antibodies (Bell *et al.*, 1997). Safar and colleagues (2005) proposed that the conformation-dependent immunoassay (CDI) be used preferentially for the tissue-based diagnosis of CJD. CDI was more sensitive (100% of 18 sCJD brain regions) compared to histology (3 of 18 [17%] of sCDJ brain regions) and immunohistochemistry (IHC) (4 of 18 [22%] of sCJD brain regions). They specifically stated that IHC *should not be used* in the diagnosis of sCJD since the CDI test was more sensitive.

Both sporadic and familial forms of CJD are currently recognized (reviewed in Kovacs *et al.*, 2005). The prion protein is encoded by the cellular gene, *PRNP*, which has been mapped to human chromosome 20p21 (Bratosiewicz *et al.*, 2004). There is positron emission tomography (PET) scan evidence in 87V-adapted scrapie Tg mice and Gerstmann–Sträussler–Scheinker (GSS) brain sections that PrP amyloid plaques can be labeled with methoxy-X04 as a possible future *in vivo* diagnostic probe in humans (Sadowski *et al.*, 2004).

Key microscopic features of a case of CJD are shown in Figure **9.4** (*Box 9.2*). Three brain lesions comprise a basic pathologic triad: severe atrophy, transcortical spongiform change, and astrocytic gliosis. This case represented the rare occurrence of clinical disease that extended over 5 years and closely mimicked the AD clinical phenotype. It underscores the need for autopsy pathologists and neurosurgeons who perform brain biopsies to be especially vigilant when examining pathologic specimens from rapidly progressive dementia patients.

Table 9.2 Simplified clinical-neuropsychological comparison of CJD vs. AD at the mild-moderate stage

Clinical profile	CJD	AD
Prevalance among dementias	Very rare	~70%
Common presenting complaints	Visual-spatial disturbances, imbalance, speech problems, mood/personality change	Forgetfulness
Neurologic/motor	Myoclonus, ataxia	Normal functioning
Neuropsychiatric	Mood disturbance, apathy, irritability, fearfulness	Depression, anxiety, delusions
Course from diagnosis to death (years)	~1	~8–10
Progression	Rapid downward decline	Gradual downward decline
Neuropsychological profile	CJD	AD
Qualitative performance differences	Variable responsiveness, perseveration, intrusion errors	Forgetfulness for instructions, receptive language problems
Confusion/disorientation	++	+
Attention/concentration deficits	+++	++
Episodic memory deficits	++	++++
Language deficits	+++	++
Executive dysfunction	+++	+++
Visual-spatial deficits	+++	+
ADL impairment	+++	++

+: relative impairment in a given cognitive-functional domain when assessed at the mild to moderate stage of disease progression. Fewer '+' signs indicate less impaired functioning. These estimates are based on neuropsychological profiles of typical/classic cases. With regards to CJD, there is insufficient data available on performance patterns in the four known subtypes (new variant, sporadic, familial, iatrogenic), and so this table focuses instead on general aspects of the disorder. The earliest manifestation of CJD may be more psychiatric or behavioral in nature, and not necessarily cognitive. Within a short period of time, however, marked cognitive deficits emerge across domains. It is important to recognize that clinical presentations of these disorders will vary across individuals, especially when different subtypes or mixed dementia pathologies are present.

(Gass *et al.*, 2000; Snowden *et al.*, 2002; Zarei *et al.*, 2002; Kapur *et al.*, 2003)

9.4 Classical features of CJD spongiform encephalopathy that include neuronal degeneration and pyknosis with striking formation of intracellular and extracellular, often confluent vacuoles. Such changes were widespread throughout the cerebrum, subcortex and hippocampus, and brainstem. Western blot analysis for pathologic prions performed at the National Prion Pathology Surveillance Center was positive. This case was unusual in having a 5-year clinical course that mimicked AD in every way. Classical signs and symptoms of sCJD were entirely absent, even in retrospect. (H&E, ×40 objective.)

Box 9.2 Histopathologic features of ALS
- Anterior horn cell loss (cervical >lumbar) in spinal cord
- Bunina bodies (2–4 µm, eosinophilic) in AHC cytoplasm or dendrites
- Skein-like inclusions (ubiquitin-positive, pNFP/SOD-1-negative, filamentous)
- Round hyaline inclusions (ubiquitin-positive, pNFP/SOD-1-negative)
- Lewy body-like hyaline inclusions (strong SOD-1 positivity)
- Axonal spheroids (Bielschowsky silver-positive)
- Basophilic inclusions (juvenile ALS marker)
- Neurofilamentous conglomerate inclusions (I113T SOD-1 mutation)
- Astrocytic hyaline inclusions (long duration SOD-1 familial ALS, SOD-1-positive)

(Kato *et al.*, 2003)

Variant CJD

The United Kingdom, especially England, experienced a major prion-associated epidemic in cattle referred to as bovine spongiform encephalopathy (BSE) (Liberski *et al.*, 1992). Thousands of infected BSE cattle were destroyed in order to control the epidemic, an approach which has been successful. However, beginning in 1997 evidence began to accumulate that BSE infectious prion agent could cross the species barrier and cause an unusual form of CJD-like illness in humans (Peden & Ironside, 2004) that is now referred to as 'variant CJD' (vCJD).

The clinical presentation, course, and duration of vCJD differ markedly from usual sCJD (Ironside *et al.*, 2003). Younger persons in their teens and 20s may be affected, psychiatric symptoms such as psychosis may be the presenting manifestation, and the course may extend beyond 1 year. The typical CJD spike pattern occurs less commonly on EEG. Ataxia, sensory symptoms with pain and dysesthesia, dysarthria, and visual abnormalities have been noted. The brain may show gross atrophy and ventricular dilatation. A peculiar type of prion-derived amyloid plaque, the 'florid plaque', is specific for vCJD. The complex plaque structure occurs when swollen degenerating synapses form 'petals' around a central compact amyloid core.

Fatal familial insomnia

Fatal familial insomnia affects sleep and waking, autonomic functions, and motor functions. Myoclonus is constant and diagnostic EEG signs of sCJD are absent (Gambetti *et al.*, 2003). Spongiform lesions that are prominent in the thalamus set this disorder apart from the pathologic expression of other prion diseases. The pathogenic mutation is substitution of aspartic acid with asparagine at codon 178, with methionine at codon 129 (D178N-129M genotype).

Gerstmann–Sträussler–Scheinkerdisease

GSS is a familial prionosis with autosomal dominant inheritance (Ghetti *et al.*, 2003). Clinically, it is characterized predominantly by slowly progressive spinocerebellar dysfunction with ataxia, absent reflexes in the legs, and cognitive impairment. Onset is usually in the fifth decade and in the early phase, ataxia is predominant (Bianca *et al.*, 2003). GSS also features deposition of tau-positive tangles that resemble AD NFTs. In addition, the cerebellum may have frequent large cored plaques composed of the aggregated prion infectious agent.

Neurofilament inclusion body disease

Recently, a new dementing 'inclusion disease' has been characterized, in which pathologically altered neurofilament subunit protein is the apparent disease-causing factor (Bigio *et al.*, 2003; Cairns & Armstrong, 2004; Cairns *et al.*, 2004a; Josephs *et al.*, 2005). An early age of onset is a very characteristic feature. Pathologic inclusions are in both neurons and glia and gray and white matter is involved. The cases have many gross and microscopic features that largely overlap with FTD tau-related disorders (see Chapter 8). The diagnosis rests on the availability of highly specific neurofilament antibodies that do not cross-react with tau antibodies. Antibodies to alpha-internexin, an intermediate filament protein, are another especially useful diagnostic marker (Cairns *et al.*, 2004b; Uchikado *et al.*, 2005).

Amyotrophic lateral sclerosis

Amyotrophic lateral sclerosis (ALS) (Lou Gehrig's disease) is the prototypical motor neuron disease with muscle wasting. Milder cognitive deficits occur in 30–50% of ALS patients; however, only a small minority of affected persons (~5%) ever become overtly demented (Swash, 2000; Kato *et al.*, 2003; Piao *et al.*, 2003; Yoshida, 2004).

Both upper and lower motor neurons may be affected and death usually results from respiratory failure and aspiration, due to impaired swallowing mechanisms. Nerve conduction abnormalities and skeletal muscle abnormalities occur (conduction velocity slowing, muscle fasciculations, 'group fiber atrophy' on muscle biopsy). Some cases (~20%) of ALS cases are familial due to a mutation of the *SOD-1* (superoxide dismutase) gene on chromosome 21. Transgenic mice (Gurney *et al.*, 1994; Doble and Kennel, 2000) and a recently developed rat model (Aoki *et al.*, 2005) carrying the human *SOD-1* transgene are widely studied to investigate the molecular pathogenic and lesion evolution in familial ALS.

Multiple clinical subtypes of ALS are recognized (Swash, 2000; Kato *et al.*, 2003; Piao *et al.*, 2003; Yoshida, 2004 for a detailed review of these syndromes). Approximately one-third of ALS patients show cognitive impairments of the FTD type (Rippon *et al.*, 2006). In one recent study, cognitive impairment was documented in 50% of 279 sporadic ALS cases (Ringholz *et al.*, 2005).

ALS microscopic features include loss of both upper (primary motor cortex, Brodmann area 4 Betz cells) and lower (spinal cord AHC) motor neurons (**9.5**). As a result, the long descending corticospinal tract nerve fibers degenerate and histologic myelin pallor (LFB-PAS stain) and axon loss (Bielschowsky silver, neurofilament antibody) can be seen in the mid-brain cerebral peduncles, the basis pontis, the medullary pyramids, and the ventral and lateral corticospinal tracts. The spinal cord anterior horns contain 2–4 µm, silver-positive inclusions called Bunina bodies and a wide variety of additional lesions (*Box 9.2*). The microscopic lesions are associated with gross atrophy of the ventral (anterior) nerve roots of the spinal cord in long-standing cases.

A biochemical link exists between ALS, motor neuron disease, and the synucleinopathies (Parkinson's disease [PD], dementia with Lewy body [DLB], and multiple systems atrophy [MSA]) and disorders with ubiquitin-positive neuronal inclusions including some cases of FTDP-17. The cytoplasm of spinal cord anterior horn motor neurons (AHC) and some neurons in the medulla and cerebral cortex may contain small, circular and discrete inclusion bodies that label strongly with antibodies to ubiquitin (Wightman *et al.*, 1992; Yoshida, 2004). Rare FTD-ALS chromosome 17q-linked cases that lack tau gene mutations have alpha-synuclein (aSYN) immunopositive inclusions (Wilhelmsen *et al.*, 2004).

Various cellular lesions and inclusions with specific immunohistochemical profiles have been characterized in sporadic and familial ALS (*Box 9.2*) (Kusaka *et al.*, 1988; Leigh *et al.*, 1988; Murayama *et al.*, 1989; Hirano, 1991; Okamoto, 1993; Kato *et al.*, 1997). Lewy body-like hyaline inclusions and astrocytic hyaline inclusions in familial ALS cases with mutations are strongly immunoreactive for SOD-1. The ubiquitin-positive AHC inclusions from a case of familial FTD-MND are illustrated in **7.27**.

9.5 A: Normal histologic appearance of human AHC. Note the large cell size, the well defined nucleolus, and clearly delineated Nissl substance and absence of vacuoles. **B**: By contrast, AHC of an FTD-ALS/MND case are fewer in number, generally smaller in size, and are slightly chromatolytic. They lack well defined Nissl substance among the brown cytoplasmic lipofuscin deposits. **C**: The primary motor cortex of the same case showed reduced numbers of all sizes of pyramidal neurons, with giant Betz cells having disappeared. Arrows point to a small cluster of surviving medium-sized motor neurons. (**A**: H&E, ×20 objective; **B**: H&E, ×25 objective; **C**: modified Bielchowsky silver, ×10 objective.)

Rare causes of acute dementia

A number of infectious and transmissible diseases can lead to acute dementia. These central nervous system (CNS) disorders include prion diseases, human immunodeficiency virus (HIV), toxoplasmosis, cryptococcus, cytomegalovirus, syphilis, borrelia, and cysticercosis (Almeida & Lautenschlager, 2005). CNS toxic and autoimmune disorders can also cause an acute-onset dementia. These latter conditions include exposure to heavy metals (lead, mercury, aluminum), carbon monoxide, and solvents (Schofield, 2005). Autoimmune causes of acute dementia include multiple sclerosis, systemic lupus erythematosus (SLE), Behçet's disease, and Sjögren's syndrome.

Causes of reversible dementia

Most screening protocols for dementia include laboratory testing to rule out hypothyoidism (Dugbartey, 1998; Davis et al., 2003) and vitamin B_{12} deficiency (Srikanth & Nagaraja, 2005) as two reversible, easily treatable causes. Normal pressure hydrocephalus (NPH) is a well recognized cause of treatable (by shunting) dementia (Srikanth and Nagaraja, 2005). Knopman and colleagues (2006) (*Box 9.3*) have called attention to cancer with or without brain metastases and chronic mental illness as important causes of nondegenerative, nonvascular dementia. Their series had no cases of NPH, subdural hematoma, hypothyroidism, vitamin B_{12} deficiency, or neurosyphilis. Cognition normalized after treatment in two individuals with acute confusion due to subdural hematoma and hypothyroidism.

Box 9.3 Nondegenerative nonvascular dementia
- 560 incident cases, 10.7% before age 70 years
- 43 cases (7.7%) were due to nondegenerative nonvascular causes
- Those 43 represented 30.0% of the total in the younger-onset group but only 5% of the over 70 age group
  - Cancer with or without brain metastases (n = 13)
  - Chronic alcoholism (n = 7)
  - Chronic mental illness (n = 11)
  - None reversed after treating the underlying cause
- No cases of dementia due to NPH, subdural hematoma, hypothyroidism, vitamin B_{12} deficiency, or neurosyphilis

(Knopman *et al.*, 2006)

There is no specific brain pathology in hypothyroidism. The pituitary glands (hypophyses) of long-standing primary thyroid-deficient individuals have a sequence of pathologic lesions (Joshi & Woolf, 2005; Khawaja *et al.*, 2006; Knopman *et al.*, 2006) that reflect the stage of the disease. The basic process reflected is an attempt by the anterior pituitary (AP) to maintain endocrine homeostasis for deficient thyroid hormones (T3, T4). In early cases, the thyrotrophs (thyroid stimulating hormone [TSH]-secreting cells of the AP) undergo simple hypertrophy and hypersecrete TSH. In middle stages of untreated hypothyroidism, TSH cells undergo hyperplasia (increase in cell number from ~5% of total AP secretory cells) and the pituitary enlarges (Alkhani *et al.*, 1999; Joshi & Woolf, 2005; Khawaja *et al.*, 2006). Thyrotrophs redistribute from their anterior medial position in the AP (Fowler & McKeel, 1979) to occupy the entire AP. The final result of years of untreated hypothyroidism is the development of nodular TSH cell AP hyperplasia, and autonomously hypersecreting TSH adenomas which may require surgical intervention. Expansion of the sella and contained pituitary gland can be easily visualized with modern neuroimaging techniques. An example of diffuse and nodular TSH hyperplasia in the AP of an untreated hypothyroid patient is shown in Figure **9.6**.

TSH hyperplasia with nonautonomous TSH adenoma formation can be reversed by treatment with thyroxin (Ashley *et al.*, 2005). Partial and complete success in thyroid hormone treatment and the degree of patient compliance with taking such medications can be judged at autopsy by assessing the size (hypertrophy), number (hyperplasia), and distribution (normal anteriomedial versus diffuse or nodular) of AP cells that secrete TSH.

9.6 A composite slide delineates the essential AP pathophysiology that accompanies clinical hypothyroidism in the absence of thyroid hormone therapy. Early TSH hyperplasia is reversible with thyroxine administration. **A**: alcian blue-positive thyrotrophs (anterior pituitary TSH cells) (Fowler & McKeel, 1979) ramifying throughout the gland rather than being confined to the anteromedial wedge. Less than 5% of normal AP cells immunostain for TSH. Within the diffusely hyperplastic gland a small round island is evident (white arrow). That TSH nodule is magnified (**B**) and thyrotrophs are labeled using an antibody to TSH-beta. The central adenomatous nodule is densely immunoreactive for TSH, while the surrounding gland shows scattered proliferated TSH cells. (**A**: Alcian blue-PAS-orange G, direct scan of histologic section; **B**: TSH-immunoperoxidase, ×1 objective.)

Box 9.4 Other neurodegenerative disorders
- Plaque-predominant and tangle-predominant variants of AD[1]
- Diffuse NFTs with calcification[2]
- Parkinsonism-dementia complex of Guam[3]
- Spinocerebellar ataxias[4]
- Friedreich's ataxia[5]
- Dentatorubral-pallidoluysian atrophy[6]
- Spinal and bulbar muscular atrophy[7]
- Iatrogenic prion disorders[8]
- Kuru[9]
- Inherited amyloidoses and neurodegeneration: familial British dementia and familial Danish dementia[10]
- Neuroaxonal dystrophies[11]
- Infantile neuroaxonal dystrophy (Seitelberger disease)[11]
- Familial encephalopathy with neuroserpin inclusion bodies[12]
- Neuronal intranuclear inclusion disease[13]

[1]Jellinger, 2003; [2]Kosaka, 1994; [3]Oyanagi, 2003; [4]Mizusawa *et al.*, 2003; [5]Robitaille *et al.*, 2003; [6]Takahashi *et al.*, 2003; [7]Sobue *et al.*, 2003; [8]Ricketts & Pergami, 2003; [9]McLean, 2003; [10]Revesz *et al.*, 2003; [11]Jellinger & Duda, 2003; [12]Davis & Collins, 2003; [13]Haltia, 2003

(From Dickson, 2003)

Multiple sclerosis (MS) cognitive impairment

Serial MRI studies can be used to assess the evolution and changing number, size, and regional CNS distribution of demyelination 'plaques' that characterize MS pathologically (Bruck & Stadelmann, 2005; Inglese *et al.*, 2005). In recent years, MRI neuroimaging also has been employed to follow cerebral atrophy as a reflection of MS disease severity (Anderson *et al.*, 2006). Diminished total cerebral cortex and brain volume may be accompanied by cognitive deficits in some MS patients. The neuropathologic basis for cerebral cortical volume loss and cognitive impairment is thought to be a result of fiber tract interruption, with loss of axonal and myelin integrity.

Increasingly, clinicians recognize that cognitive impairment is an important part of the expression of MS (Denney *et al.*, 2004; Calabrese, 2006). In one study, for example, 31% of MS patients had some cognitive deficit that was judged as mild in 15%, moderate in 11.2%, and severe in 4.8% (Nocentini *et al.*, 2006).

Other disorders

Certain other neurodegenerative and dementing disease entities could not be addressed due to space and time limitations. They are included for completeness as a guide to interested readers (see *Box 9.4*).

Table 9.1 references

HS

Ala *et al.*, 2000; Barker *et al.*, 2002; Blass *et al.*, 2003; Corey-Bloom et al., 1997; Dickson *et al.*, 1994; Fish & Spencer, 1995; Hatanpaa *et al.*, 2004; Mintzer *et al.*, 2004; Petersen *et al.*, 2006.

Nucleotide repeat disorders: HD

Andrews*et al.*, 1999; Aylward *et al.*, 2000; Hedreen *et al.*, 1991; Heinsen *et al.*, 1994; Huntington's Disease Collaborative Research Group, The , 1993; Persichetti *et al.*, 1994; Sapp *et al.*, 1997; Sotrel *et al.*, 1991; Vonsattel *et al.*, 1985; Xuereb *et al.*, 1996.

Kuf's disease (ceroid lipofuscinosis)

Josephson *et al.*, 2001; Mole *et al.*, 2005.

Prion diseases (CJD, vCJD, FFI, GSS, kuru, BSE)

Bell *et al.*, 1997; Bianca *et al.*, 2003; Bratosiewicz-Wasik *et al.*, 2004; Budka *et al.*, 2003; Carleton Gajdusek, 1977 Chakraborty *et al.*, 2005; Cooper *et al.*, 2005; Gambetti *et al.*, 2003; Gambetti *et al.*, 2003; Ghetti *et al.*, 2003; http://www.cjdsurveillance.com (website link); Ironside *et al.*, 2003; Ishida *et al.*, 2005; Klug *et al.*, 2005; Kovacs *et al.*, 2005; Lee *et al.*, 2005; Liberski *et al.*, 1992; Peden & Ironside, 2004; Priola *et al.*, 2006; Sadowski *et al.*, 2004; Safar *et al.*, 2005; Safar *et al.*, 2005; Stephenson, 1997; Van Everbroeck *et al.*, 2000.

Neurofilament inclusion body disease

Bigio *et al.*, 2003; Cairns & Armstrong, 2004; Cairns *et al.*, 2004, b; Josephs *et al.*, 2005; Uchikado *et al.*, 2005.

ALS

Aoki *et al.*, 2005; Doble & Kennel, 2000; Gurney *et al.*, 1994; Hirano, 1991; Kato *et al.*, 1997; Kato *et al.*, 2003; Kusaka *et al.*, 1988; Leigh *et al.*, 1988; Murayama *et al.*, 1989; Okamoto, 1993; Piao *et al.*, 2003; Ringholz *et al.*, 2005; Rippon *et al.*, 2006; Swash, 2000; Wightman *et al.*, 1992; Wilhelmsen *et al.*, 2004; Yoshida, 2004.

Rare causes of acute dementia

Almeida & Lautenschlager, 2005; Schofield, 2005.

Causes of reversible dementia

Alkhani *et al.*, 1999; Ashley *et al.*, 2005; Davis *et al.*, 2003; Dugbartey, 1998; Fowler & McKeel, 1979; Joshi & Woolf, 2005; Khawaja *et al.*, 2006; Knopman *et al.*, 2006; Srikanth & Nagaraja, 2005.

Multiple sclerosis: cognitive impairment

Anderson *et al.*, 2006; Bruck & Stadelmann, 2005; Calabrese, 2006; Denney *et al.*, 2004; Inglese *et al.*, 2005; Nocentini *et al.*, 2006.

References

Ala TA, Beh GO, Frey WH, II (2000). Pure hippocampal sclerosis: a rare cause of dementia mimicking Alzheimer's disease. *Neurology* 54:843–848.

Alkhani AM, Cusimano M, Kovacs K, *et al.* (1999). Cytology of pituitary thyrotroph hyperplasia in protracted primary hypothyroidism. *Pituitary* 1:291–295.

Almeida OP, Lautenschlager NT (2005). Dementia associated with infectious diseases. *Int. Psychogeriatr.* **17** (Suppl 1):S65–S77.

Anderson VM, Fox NC, Miller DH (2006). Magnetic resonance imaging measures of brain atrophy in multiple sclerosis. *J. Magn. Reson. Imaging* 23:605–618.

Andrews TC, Weeks RA, Turjanski RN, *et al.* (1999). Huntington's disease progression. PET and clinical observations. *Brain* 122:2353–2356.

Aoki M, Kato S, Nagai M, Itoyama Y (2005). Development of a rat model of amyotrophic lateral sclerosis expressing a human SOD-1 transgene. *Neuropathology* 25:365–370.

Ashley WW Jr, Ojemann JG, Park TS, *et al.* (2005). Primary hypothyroidism in a 12-year-old girl with a suprasellar pituitary mass: rapid regression after thyroid replacement therapy: case report. *J. Neurosurg.* 102(4 Suppl):413–416.

Awano T, Katz ML, O'Brien DP, *et al.* (2006). A frame shift mutation in canine TPP1 (the ortholog of human CLN2) in a juvenile Dachshund with neuronal ceroid lipofuscinosis. *Mol. Genet. Metab.* Apr 16 (e-publication).

Aylward EH, Codori AM, Rosenblatt A, *et al.* (2000). Rate of caudate atrophy in presymptomatic and symptomatic stages of Huntington's disease. *Mov. Disord.* **15**:552–560.

Barker WW, Luis CA, Kashuba A, *et al.* (2002). Relative frequencies of Alzheimer disease, Lewy body, vascular and frontotemporal dementia, and hippocampal sclerosis in the State of Florida Brain Bank. *Alz. Dis. Assoc. Disord.* **16**:203–212.

Bell JE, Gentleman SM, Ironside JW, *et al.* (1997). Prion protein immunocytochemistry: UK five centre consensus report. *Neuropathol. Appl. Neurobiol.* **23**:26–35.

Bianca M, Bianca S, Vecchio I, *et al.* (2003). Gerstmann–Sträussler–Scheinker disease with P102L-V129 mutation: a case with psychiatric manifestations at onset. *Annales de Genetique* **46**:467–469.

Bigio EH, Lipton AM, White CL 3rd, *et al.* (2003). Frontotemporal and motor neurone degeneration with neurofilament inclusion bodies: additional evidence for overlap between FTD and ALS. *Neuropathol. Appl. Neurobiol.* **29**:239–253.

Blass DM, Hatanpaa KJ, Brandt J, *et al.* (2003). Dementia in hippocampal sclerosis resembles frontotemporal dementia more than Alzheimer's disease. *Neurology* **63**:492–497.

Bonsignore M, Tessa A, Rosa GD, *et al.* (2006). Novel CLN1 mutation in two Italian sibs with late infantile neuronal ceroid lipofuscinosis. *Eur. J. Paediatr. Neurol.* Jun 5 (e-publication).

Bratosiewicz-Wasik J, Wasik TJ, Liberski PP (2004). Molecular approaches to mechanisms of prion diseases. [Review] [92 refs] *Folia Neuropathol.* **42** (Suppl A):33–46.

Bruck W, Stadelmann C (2005). The spectrum of multiple sclerosis: new lessons from pathology. *Curr. Opin. Neurol.* **18**:221–224.

Budka H, Head MW, Ironside JW, *et al.* (2003). Chapter 6. Prion disorders: sporadic Creutzfeldt-Jakob disease. In: *Neurodegeneration: The Molecular Pathology of Dementia and Movement Disorders.* DW Dickson (ed). ISN Neuropath Press, Basel, pp. 287–297.

Cairns NJ, Armstrong RA (2004). Quantification of the pathological changes in the temporal lobe of patients with a novel neurofilamentopathy: neurofilament inclusion disease (NID). *Clin. Neuropathol.* **23**:107–112.

Cairns NJ, Grossman M, Arnold SE, *et al.* (2004a). Clinical and neuropathologic variation in neuronal intermediate filament inclusion disease. *Neurology* **63**:1376–1384.

Cairns NJ, Uryu K, Bigio EH, *et al.* (2004b). Alpha-internexin aggregates are abundant in neuronal intermediate filament inclusion disease (NIFID) but rare in other neurodegenerative diseases. *Acta Neuropathol.* (Berl) **108**:213–223.

Calabrese P (2006). Neuropsychology of multiple sclerosis: an overview. *J. Neurol.* **253** (Suppl 1):I10–I15.

Cannelli N, Cassandrini D, Bertini E, *et al.* (2006). Novel mutations in CLN8 in Italian variant late infantile neuronal ceroid lipofuscinosis: another genetic hit in the Mediterranean. *Neurogenetics* 7(2):111–117.

D Carleton Gajdusek, MD-Noble Laureate in Medicine for 1976 (1977). *Arch. Neurol.* **34**:205–208.

Chakraborty C, Nandi S, Jana S (2005). Prion disease: a deadly disease for protein misfolding. [Review] [111 refs] *Curr. Pharm. Biotech.* **6**:167–177.

Collins J, Holder GE, Herbert H, *et al.* (2006). Batten disease: features to facilitate early diagnosis. *Br. J. Ophthalmol.* Jun 5 (e-publication).

Cooper SA, Murray KL, Heath CA, Will RG, Knight RS (2005). Isolated visual symptoms at onset in sporadic Creutzfeldt-Jakob disease: the clinical phenotype of the 'Heidenhain variant'. *Br. J. Ophthalmol.* **89**:1341–1342.

Corey-Bloom J, Sabbagh MN, Bondi MW, *et al.* (1997). Hippocampal sclerosis contributes to dementia in the elderly. *Neurology* **48**:154–160.

Davis JD, Stern RA, Flashman LA (2003). Cognitive and neuropsychiatric aspects of subclinical hypothyroidism: significance in the elderly. [Review] *Curr. Psychiatry Rep.* **5**:384–390.

Davis R, Collins GH (2003). Chapter 9. Other neurodegenerative disorders: familial encephalopathy with neuroserpin inclusion bodies. In: *Neurodegeneration: The Molecular Pathology of Dementia and Movement Disorders.* DW Dickson (ed). ISN Neuropath Press, Basel, pp. 400–403.

Denney DR, Lynch SG, Parmenter BA, *et al.* (2004). Cognitive impairment in relapsing and primary progressive multiple sclerosis: mostly a matter of speed. *J. Int. Neuropsychol. Soc.* **10**:948–956.

Dickson DW (ed) (2003). *Neurodegeneration: The Molecular Pathology of Dementia and Movement Disorders.* ISN Neuropath Press, Basel.

Dickson DW, Davies P, Bevona C, *et al.* (1994). Hippocampal sclerosis: a common pathological feature of dementia in very old (> or = 80 years of age) humans. *Acta Neuropathol.* **88**:212–221.

Doble A, Kennel P (2000). Animal models of amyotrophic lateral sclerosis. *Amyotroph. Lateral Scler. Other Motor Neuron Disord.* **1**:301–312.

Dugbartey AT (1998). Neurocognitive aspects of hypothyroidism. *Arch. Intern. Med.* **158**:1413–1418.

Fish DR, Spencer SS (1995). Clinical correlations: MRI and EEG. [Review] *Magn. Reson. Imaging* **13**:1113–1117.

Fowler MR, McKeel DW Jr (1979). Human adenohypophyseal quantitative histochemical cell classification. I. Morphologic criteria and cell type distribution. *Arch. Pathol. Lab. Med.* **103**:613–620.

Gambetti P, Kong Q, Zou W, *et al.* (2003). Sporadic and familial CJD: classification and characterisation. *Br. Med. Bull.* **66**:213–239.

Gambetti P, Parchi P, Chen SG, *et al.* (2003). Chapter 6. Prion disorders: fatal insomnia: familial and sporadic. In: *Neurodegeneration: The Molecular Pathology of Dementia and Movement Disorders.* DW Dickson (ed). ISN Neuropath Press, Basel, pp. 326–332.

Gass CS, Luis CA, Meyers TL, *et al.* (2000). Familial Creutzfeldt-Jakob disease: a neuropsychological case study. *Arch. Clin. Neuropsychol.* **15**(2):165–175.

Ghetti B, Bugiani O, Tagliavini F, *et al.* (2003). Chapter 6. Prion disorders: Gerstmann–Sträussler–Scheinker disease. In: *Neurodegeneration: The Molecular Pathology of Dementia and Movement Disorders.* DW Dickson (ed). ISN Neuropath Press, Basel, pp. 318–325.

Gurney ME Pu H, Chiu AY, *et al.* (1994). Motor neuron degenration in mice that express a human Cu,Zn superoxide dismutase mutation. *Science* **264**:1772–1775.

Haltia M (2003). Chapter 9. Other neurodegenerative disorders: neuronal intranuclear inclusion disease. In: *Neurodegeneration: The Molecular Pathology of Dementia and Movement Disorders.* DW Dickson (ed). ISN Neuropath Press, Basel, pp. 404–406.

Hatanpaa KJ, Blass DM, Pletnikova O, *et al.* (2004). Most cases of dementia with hippocampal sclerosis may represent frontotemporal dementia. *Neurology* **63**:538–542.

Hedreen JC, Peyser CE, Folstein SE, *et al.* (1991). Neuronal loss in layers V and VI of cerebral cortex in Huntington's disease. *Neurosci. Lett.* **133**:257–261.

Heinsen H, Strik M, Bauer M, *et al.* (1994). Cortical and striatal neurone number in Huntington's disease. *Acta Neuropathol.* **88**:320–333.

Hirano A (1991). Cytopathology of amyotrophic lateral sclerosis. *Adv. Neurol.* **58**:901–910.

Huntington's Disease Collaborative Research Group (1993). A novel gene containing a trinucleotide repeat that is expanded and unstable on Huntington's disease chromosomes. *Cell* **72**:971–983.

Inglese M, Grossman RI, Filippi M (2005). Magnetic resonance imaging monitoring of multiple sclerosis lesion evolution. [Review] *J. Neuroimaging* **15**(4 Suppl):22S–29S.

Ironside JW, Head MW, Will RG (2003). Chapter 6. Prion disorders: variant Creutzfeldt-Jakob disease. In: *Neurodegeneration: The Molecular Pathology of Dementia and Movement Disorders.* DW Dickson (ed). ISN Neuropath Press, Basel, pp. 310–317.

Ishida C, Okino S, Kitamoto T, *et al.* (2005). Involvement of the peripheral nervous system in human prion diseases including dural graft associated Creutzfeldt-Jakob disease. *J. Neurol. Neurosurg. Psychiatr.* **76**:325–329.

Jellinger K (2003). Chapter 2. Alzheimer's disease and ageing: plaque-predominant and tangle-predominant variants of AD. In: *Neurodegeneration: The Molecular Pathology of Dementia and Movement Disorders.* DW Dickson (ed). ISN Neuropath Press, Basel, pp. 66–68.

Jellinger K, Duda J (2003). Chapter 9. Other neurodegenerative disorders: neuroaxonal dystrophies. In: *Neurodegeneration: The Molecular Pathology of Dementia and Movement Disorders.* DW Dickson (ed). ISN Neuropath Press, Basel, pp. 386–393.

Josephs KA, Uchikado H, McComb RD, *et al.* (2005). Extending the clinicopathological spectrum of neurofilament inclusion disease. *Acta Neuropathol.* (Berl) **109**:427–432.

Josephson SA, Schmidt RE, Millsap P, *et al.* (2001). Autosomal dominant Kufs' disease: a cause of early onset dementia. *J. Neurol. Sci.* **188**:51–60.

Joshi AS, Woolf PD (2005). Pituitary hyperplasia secondary to primary hypothyroidism: a case report and review of the literature. *Pituitary* **8**:99–103.

Kapur N, Abbott P, Lowman A, *et al.* (2003). The neuropsychological profile associated with variant Creutzfeld-Jacob disease. *Brain* **126**:2693–2702.

Kato S, Hayashi H, Nakashima K, *et al.* (1997). Pathological characterization of astrocytic hyaline inclusions in familial amyotrophic lateral sclerosis. *Am. J. Pathol.* **151**:611–620.

Kato S, Shaw P, Wood-Alum C, *et al.* (2003). Chapter 8. Motor neurone disorders: amyotrophic lateral sclerosis. In: *Neurodegeneration: The Molecular Pathology of Dementia and Movement Disorders.* DW Dickson (ed). ISN Neuropath Press, Basel, pp. 350–368.

Khawaja NM, Taher BM, Barham ME, *et al.* (2006). Pituitary enlargement in patients with primary hypothyroidism. *Endocr. Pract.* **12**:29–34.

Klug GM, Boyd A, Lewis V, *et al.* (2005). Creutzfeldt-Jakob disease: Australian surveillance update to 31 December 2004. [Review] [3 refs] *Comm. Dis. Intell.* **29**:269–271.

Knopman DS, Petersen RC, Cha RH, *et al.* (2006). Incidence and causes of nondegenerative nonvascular dementia: a population-based study. *Arch. Neurol.* **63**:218–221.

Kosaka K (1994). Diffuse neurofibrillary tangles with calcification: a new presenile dementia. *J. Neurol. Neurosurg. Psychiatr.* **57**:594–596.

Kovacs GG, Puopolo M, Ladogana A, *et al.* (2005). Genetic prion disease: the EUROCJD experience. *Human Genetics* **118**:166–174.

Kusaka H, Imai T, Hashimoto S, *et al.* (1988). Ultrastructural study of chromatolytic neurons in an adult-onset sporadic case of amyotrophic lateral sclerosis. *Acta Neuropathol.* **75**:523–528.

Lee CC, Kuo LT, Wang CH, *et al.* (2005). An SF. Accumulation of prion protein in the peripheral nervous system in human prion diseases. *J. Neuropath. Exp. Neurol.* **64**:716–721.

Leigh PN, Anderton BH, Dodson A, *et al.* (1988). Ubiquitin deposits in anterior horn cells in motor neurone disease. *Neurosci. Lett.* **93**:197–203.

Liberski PP, Yanagihara R, Wells GA, *et al.* (1992). Comparative ultrastructural neuropathology of naturally occurring bovine spongiform encephalopathy and experimentally induced scrapie and Creutzfeldt-Jakob disease. *J. Comp. Pathol.* **106**:361–381.

McLean CA (2003). Chapter 6. Prion disorders: Kuru. In: *Neurodegeneration: The Molecular Pathology of Dementia and Movement Disorders.* DW Dickson (ed). ISN Neuropath Press, Basel, pp. 333–334.

Mintzer S, Cendes F, Soss J, *et al.* (2004). Unilateral hippocampal sclerosis with contralateral temporal scalp ictal onset. *Epilepsia* **45**:792–802.

Mizusawa H, Clark HB, Koeppen AH (2003). Chapter 5. Trinucleotide repeat disorders: spinocerebellar ataxias. In: *Neurodegeneration: The Molecular Pathology of Dementia and Movement Disorders.* DW Dickson (ed). ISN Neuropath Press, Basel, pp. 242–256.

Mole SE, Williams RE, Goebel HH (2005). Correlations between genotype, ultrastructural morphology and clinical phenotype in the neuronal ceroid lipofuscinoses. [Review] *Neurogenetics* **6**:107–126.

Murayama S, Ookawa Y, Mori H, *et al.* (1989). Immunocytochemical and ultrastructural study of Lewy body-like hyaline inclusions in familial amyotrophic lateral sclerosis. *Acta Neuropathol.* **78**:143–152.

Nocentini U, Pasqualetti P, Bonavita S, *et al.* (2006). Cognitive dysfunction in patients with relapsing-remitting multiple sclerosis. *Mult. Scler.* **12**:77–87.

Okamoto K (1993). Bunina bodies in amyotrophic lateral sclerosis. *Neuropathology* **13**:193–199.

Oyanagi K (2003). Chapter 3. Tauopathies: parkinsonism-dementia complex of Guam. In: *Neurodegeneration: The Molecular Pathology of Dementia and Movement Disorders.* DW Dickson (ed). ISN Neuropath Press, Basel, pp. 137–142.

Peden AH, Ironside JW (2004). Review: pathology of variant Creutzfeldt-Jakob disease. *Folia Neuropathol.* **42** (Suppl A):85–91.

Persichetti F, Srinidhi J, Kanaley L, *et al.* (1994). Huntington's disease CAG trinucleotide repeats in pathologically confirmed postmortem brains. *Neurobiol. Dis.* **1**:159–166.

Petersen RC, Parisi JE, Dickson DW, *et al.* (2006). Neuropathologic features of amnestic mild cognitive impairment. *Arch. Neurol.* **63**:665–672.

Piao Y-S, Wakabayashi K, Kakita A, *et al.* (2003). Neuropathology with clinical correlations of sporadic amyotrophic lateral sclerosis: 102 autopsy cases examined between 1962 and 2000. *Brain Pathol.* **12**:10–22.

Priola SA, Vorberg I (2006). Molecular aspects of disease pathogenesis in the transmissible spongiform encephalopathies. *Mol. Biotechnol.* **33**:71–88.

Revesz T, Ghiso J, Plant GT, *et al.* (2003). Chapter 9. Other neurodegenerative disorders: inherited amyloidoses and neurodegeneration: familial British dementia and familial Danish dementia. In: *Neurodegeneration: The Molecular Pathology of Dementia and Movement Disorders.* DW Dickson (ed). ISN Neuropath Press, Basel, pp. 380–385.

Ricketts MN, Pergami P (2003). Chapter 6. Prion disorders: iatrogenic prion disorders. In: *Neurodegeneration: The Molecular Pathology of Dementia and Movement Disorders.* DW Dickson (ed). ISN Neuropath Press, Basel, pp. 307–309.

Ringholz GM, Appel SH, Bradshaw M, *et al.* (2005). Prevalence and patterns of cognitive impairment in sporadic ALS. *Neurology* **65**:586–590.

Rippon GA, Scarmeas N, Gordon PH, *et al.* (2006). An observational study of cognitive impairment in amyotrophic lateral sclerosis. *Arch. Neurol.* **63**:319–320.

Robitaille Y, Klockgether T, Lamarche JB (2003). Chapter 5. Trinucleotide repeat disorders: Friedreich's ataxia. In: *Neurodegeneration: The Molecular Pathology of Dementia and Movement Disorders.* DW Dickson (ed). ISN Neuropath Press, Basel, pp. 257–268.

Sadowski M, Pankiewicz J, Scholtzova H, *et al.* (2004). Targeting prion amyloid deposits in vivo. *J. Neuropath. Exp. Neurol.* **63**:775–784.

Safar JG, Geschwind MD, Deering C, *et al.* (2005). Diagnosis of human prion disease. *Proc. Natl. Acad. Sci. USA* **102**:3501–3506.

Sapp E, Schwarz C, Chase K, *et al.* (1997). Huntingtin localization in brains of normal and Huntington's disease brains. *Ann. Neurol.* **42**:604–612.

Schofield P (2005). Dementia associated with toxic causes and autoimmune disease. *Int. Psychogeriatr.* **17** (Suppl 1):S129–147.

Schulz A, Mousallem T, Venkataramani M, *et al.* (2006).The CLN9 protein, a regulator of dihydroceramide synthase. *J. Biol. Chem.* **281**(5):2784–2794.

Seehafer SS, Pearce DA (2006). You say lipofuscin, we say ceroid: defining autofluorescent storage material. *Neurobiol. Aging* **27**(4):576–588.

Siintola E, Topcu M, Kohlschutter A, *et al.* (2005). Two novel CLN6 mutations in variant late-infantile neuronal ceroid lipofuscinosis patients of Turkish origin. *Clin. Genet.* **68**(2):167–173.

Snowden JS, Mann DMA, Neary D (2002). Distinct neuropsychological characteristics in Creutzfeldt-Jakob disease. *J. Neurol. Neurosurg. Psychiatr.* **73**:686–694.

Sobue G, Adachi H, Katsuno M (2003). Chapter 5. Trinucleotide repeat disorders: spinal and bulbar muscular atrophy. In: *Neurodegeneration: The Molecular Pathology of Dementia and Movement Disorders.* DW Dickson (ed). ISN Neuropath Press, Basel, pp. 275–279.

Sotrel A, Paskevich PA, Kiely DK, *et al.* (1991). Morphometric analysis of the prefrontal cortex in Huntington's disease. *Neurology* **41**:1117–1123.

Srikanth S, Nagaraja AV (2005). A prospective study of reversible dementias: frequency, causes, clinical profile, and results of treatment. *Neurol. India* **53**(3):291–294; discussion 294–296.

Stephenson J (1997). Nobel Prize to Stanley Prusiner for prion discovery. *JAMA* **278**:1479.

Swash M (2000). Clinical features and diagnosis of amyotrophic lateral sclerosis. In: *Amyotrophic Lateral Sclerosis.* RH Brown, V Meininger, M Swash (eds). Martin Dunitz, London, pp. 3–30.

Takahashi H, Yamada M, Tsuji S (2003). Chapter 5. Trinucleotide repeat disorders: dentatorubral-pallidoluysian atrophy. In: *Neurodegeneration: The Molecular Pathology of Dementia and Movement Disorders.* DW Dickson (ed). ISN Neuropath Press, Basel, pp. 269–274.

Uchikado H, Shaw G, Wang DS, *et al.* (2005). Screening for neurofilament inclusion disease using alpha-internexin immunohistochemistry. *Neurology* **64**:1658–1659.

Van Everbroeck B, Pals P, Dziedzic T, *et al.* (2000). Retrospective study of Creutzfeldt-Jakob disease in Belgium: neuropathological findings. *Acta Neuropathol. (Berl)* **99**:358–364.

Vonsattel JP, Myers RH, Stevens TJ, *et al.* (1985). Neuropathological classification of Huntington's disease. *J. Neuropathol. Exp. Neurol.* **44**:559–577.

Wightman G, Anderson VE, Martin J, *et al.* (1992). Hippocampal and neocortical ubiquitin-immunoreactive inclusions in amyotrophic lateral sclerosis with dementia. *Neurosci. Lett.* **139**:269–274.

Wilhelmsen KC, Forman MS, Rosen HJ, *et al.* (2004). 17q-linked frontotemporal dementia-amyotrophic lateral sclerosis without tau mutations with tau and alpha-synuclein inclusions. *Arch. Neurol.* **61**:398–340.

Xuereb JH, MacMillan JC, Snell R, *et al.* (1996). Neuropathological diagnosis and CAG repeat expansion in Huntington's disease. *J. Neurol. Neurosurg. Psychiatr.* **60**:78–81.

Yoshida M (2004). Amyotrophic lateral sclerosis with dementia: the clinicopathological spectrum. *Neuropathology* **24**:87–102.

Zarei M, Nouraei SAR, Caine D, *et al.* (2002). Neuropsychological and quantitative oculometric study of a case of sporadic Creutzfeldt-Jakob disease at pre-dementia stage. *J. Neurol. Neurosurg. Psychiatr.* **73**:56–58.

Appendix

ADRC Washington University School of Medicine: Bielschowsky-MBT (for tangles)

20% silver nitrate
20 g silver nitrate add to
100 ml DH2O, stir to dissolve

Ammoniacal silver
Add vacuumed ammonia to 20% silver drop by drop until the solution gets cloudy then turns clear, filter before use

5% Hypo
5 g sodium thiosulfate
100 ml DH2O mix and dissolve

Developer
100 ml DH2O
20 ml 35% formaldehyde
0.5 g citric acid
1 drop nitric acid, mix and dissolve in order

1 Hydrate slides to DH2O and rinse for 5 minutes.
2 Impregnate slides in 20% silver nitrate for 20 minutes at room temperature.
3 Rinse in DH2O approximately 5 minutes.
4 Pour the ammonical silver solution (filtered) on the slides and let it sit for 15 minutes.
5 Pour the ammonical silver solution into a clean container; wash the slides in a weak ammonia solution for 3–5 minutes.
6 Add 3 drops of developer per 100 ml silver solution. Stir.
7 Pour off the wash solution and pour on the developer solution. Developing takes 5–10 minutes (watch carefully).
8 Rinse in DH2O for about 5 minutes.
9 Place in hypo solution for 30 seconds to 3 minutes; watch until it turns a nice brown color.
10 Rinse in DH2O for 3–5 minutes, then dehydrate back to xylene, coverslip.

Notes
1 *Always* acid clean your dishes.
2 *Never* use metal in silver solutions.
3 *Always* wear gloves when using silver – it will develop on your skin.
4 *Always* use fresh reagents.
5 Use powder-free gloves only.
6 Place ammonia on vacuum for 20 minutes.

Materials needed
1 Silver nitrate – EMS #21052
2 Sodium thiosulfate – Fisher # AC20287-5000
3 Citric acid – Sigma C7129

ADRC Washington University School of Medicine: hematoxylin and eosin (H&E)

1 Run the slide down to DH2O.
2 Place in hematoxylin for 10 minutes.
3 Rinse in DH2O for 5 minutes, 1 dip in acid alcohol, wash in DH2O, 8 dips in ammonia water, wash in DH2O for 15 minutes.
4 Dip 1–3 times in 95% alcohol.
5 Place in eosin for 3 minutes.
6 Wash in DH2O for 3–5 minutes.
7 Quickly run down to xylene and coverslip.

Notes
1 Use the ThermoShandon Instant Hematoxylin and Eosin with phyloxine for this stain protocol (2/13/02) order #6765015.
2 Follow the protocol in the AFIP *Staining Manual* to make eosin with phyloxine.

Further reading

Baker M, Mackenzie IR, Pickering-Brown SM, *et al.* (2006). Mutations in progranulin cause tau-negative frontotemporal dementia linked to chromosome 17. *Nature* **442**:916–919.

Chapter 3

Dickson DW (2005). Required techniques and useful molecular markers in the neuropathologic diagnosis of neurodegenerative diseases. [Review] [86 refs] *Acta Neuropathol.* **109**:14–24.

Halliday G, Ng T, Rodriguez M, *et al.* (2002). Consensus neuropathological diagnosis of common dementia syndromes: testing and standardizing the use of multiple diagnostic criteria. *Acta Neuropathol.* 104:72–78.

Knopman DS, Boeve BF, Petersen RC (2003). Essentials of the proper diagnoses of mild cognitive impairment, dementia, and major subtypes of dementia. *Mayo Clin. Proc.* **78**:1290–1308.

Schmitz C, Hof PR (2005). Design-based stereology in neuroscience. [Review] [120 refs] *Neuroscience* **130**:813–831.

Chapter 4

Braak H, Braak E (1997). Frequency of stages of Alzheimer-related lesions in different age categories. *Neurobiol. Aging* **18**:351–357.

Terman A, Brunk UT (2004). Aging as a catabolic malfunction. [Review] [101 refs] *Inter. J. Biochem. Cell Biol.* **236**:2365–2375.

Chapter 5

Petersen RC, Parisi JE, Dickson DW *et al.* (206). Neuropathologic features of amnestic mild cognitive impairment. *Arch. Neurol.* **63**:665–672.

Chapter 6

Akopov S, Sercombe R, Seylaz J (1996). Cerebrovascular reactivity: role of endothelium/platelet/leukocyte interactions. [Review] [432 refs] *Cerebrovascular Brain Metabol. Reviews* **8**:11–94.

Choi JY, Morris JC, Hsu CY (1998). Aging and cerebrovascular disease [Review]. *Neurol. Clinics* **16** (3):687–711.

Chapter 7

Chin SS-M, Goldman JE (1996). Glial inclusions in CNS degenerative diseases. *J. Neuropathol. Exp. Neurobiol.* **55**:499–508.

Dev KK, Hofele K, Barbieri S *et al.* (2003). Part II: Alpha-synuclein and its molecular pathophysiological role in neurodegenerative disease. [Review] [402 refs] *Neuropharmacol.* **45**(1):14–44.

Hashimoto M, Rockenstein E, Masliah E (2003). Transgenic models of alpha-synuclein pathology: past, present, and future. [Review] [82 refs] *Ann. N. Y. Acad. Sci.* **991**:171–188.

Jellinger KA (2003). Neuropathological spectrum of synucleinopathies. [Review] [77 refs] *Movement Dis.* **18**(Suppl 6):S2-S12

Norris EH, Giasson BI, Lee VM (2004). Alpha-synuclein: normal function and role in neurodegenerative diseases. [Review] [253 refs] *Curr. Top. Develop. Biol.* **60**:17–54.

Roy CN, Andrews NC (2001). Recent advances in disorders of iron metabolism: mutations, mechanisms and modifiers. [Review] [62 refs] *Human Molecular Genetics* **10**(20):2181–2186.

Sadrzadeh SM, Saffari Y (2004). Iron and brain disorders. [Review] [84 refs] *Am. J. Clin. Pathol.* **121**(Suppl):S64–S70.

Chapter 8

Assal F, Cummings JL (2002). Neuropsychiatric symptoms in the dementias. [Review] [56 refs] *Curr. Opin. Neurol.* **15**(4):445–450.

Cairns NJ, Lee VM, Trojanowski JQ (2004). The cytoskeleton in neurodegenerative diseases. [Review] [126 refs] *J. Pathol.* **204**(4):438–449.

Eckert T, Barnes A, Dhawan V *et al.* (2005). FDG PET in the differential diagnosis of parkinsonian disorders. *Neuroimage* **26**(3):912–921.

Ferrer I, Gomez-Isla T, Puig B *et al.* (2005). Current advances on different kinases involved in tau phosphorylation, and implications in Alzheimer's disease and tauopathies. [Review] [144 refs] *Curr. Alz. Res.* **2**(1):3–18.

Ingelsson M, Hyman BT (2002). Disordered proteins in dementia. [Review] [150 refs] *Ann. Med.* **34**(4):259–271.

Knopman DS, Boeve BS, Petersen RC (2003). Essentials of the proper diagnoses of mild cognitive impairment, dementia, and major subtypes of dementia. *Mayo Clin. Proc.* **78**:1290–1308.

Lang AE (2005). Treatment of progressive supranuclear palsy and corticobasal degeneration. *Movement Dis.* **20**(Suppl 12):S83–S91.

Lewis J, Dickson DW (2003). Transgenic animal models of tauopathy. In: Dickson DW, *Neurodegeneration: The Molecular Pathology of Dementia and Movement Disorders*, ISN Neuropath Press, Basel, pp. 150–154.

Sergeant N, Delacourte A, Buee L (2005). Tau protein as a differential biomarker of tauopathies. [Review] [249 refs] *Biochimica et Biophysica Acta* **1739**(2–3):179–197.

Snowden JS, Neary D, Mann DMA (1996). *Frontotemporal Lobar Dementia: Fronto-temporal Dementia, Progressive Aphasia, Semantic Dementia*. Churchill Livingstone, New York.

National Alzheimer's Coordinating Center (NACC)

Headquarters: University of Washington, Seattle.

Principal Investigator: Walter A Kukull, PhD Epidemiology, University of Washington.

Funding source: National Institute on Aging (NIA), Bethesda, MD.

Research projects: UDS Database (Uniform Data Set), Collaborative research grants, Methodological research grants, involving Alzheimer Disease Centers (ADCs).

Activities: To perform required administrative functions: logistical support for Directors and Core Leaders meetings, interface with NIA 'initiative' groups; provide distribution of funds in support of NACC data collection effort and Collaborative Projects; and inter-ADC communication and other affiliated activities.

Contact information:
- Telephone: (206) 543-8637
- Fax: (206) 616-5927
- E-mail: naccmail@u.Washington.edu
- Website: http://www.alz.Washington.edu/
- Mail address: 4311 11th Ave NE, #300, Seattle, WA 98105, USA

National Diabetes Research Interchange (NDRI)

Headquarters: Philadelphia, Pennsylvania.

Principal Investigator: D Walter Cohen, DDS, Chairman, Chancellor Emeritus, Drexel University College of Medicine, Philadelphia, PA, is Chairman of the Board of Directors with more than 60 scientists on various NDRI subcommittees.

Funding source: National Institutes of Health, Bethesda, MD; Juvenile Diabetes Association; NDRI Partners Program, voluntary health organizations and private donations.

Research projects: Database, human tissue bank distribution for research (Human Tissue and Organs for Research Program), The Human Biological Data Interchange (HBDI) database and pedigree catalog.

Activities: Sponsors conferences on use of human tissues for research. Facilitates use of human tissues in diabetes and other types of human disorders research.

Contact information:
- Telephone: (800) 222-NDRI (6374) or (215) 557-7361
- Fax: (215) 557-7154
- E-mail: info@ndriresource.org
- Website: http://www.ndriresource.org; http://www.ndri.com
- Mail address: 8 Penn Center, 8th Floor, 1628 JFK Boulevard, Philadelphia, PA 19103-2125, USA

National Prion Disease Pathology Surveillance Center

Headquarters: Case Western University, Cleveland, Ohio

Principal Investigator: Pierluigi Gambetti, M.D., Director, Bernardino Ghetti, Co-Director

Funding source: National Institute on Aging (NIA), Bethesda, MD

Mission: Provide surveillance for prion disorders, including variant Creutzfeldt-Jacob disease (vCJD); detect species jumping of Bovine Spongiform Encephalitis (BSE) from cattle to man

Purposes of the Center:

• Acquire tissue samples and clinical information from as many cases of human prion disease occurring in the United States as possible in order to help monitor the possible occurrence of variant CJD (vCJD) in the USA.

• Help establish the diagnosis of prion disease by analyzing cerebrospinal fluid (CSF), blood, and brain tissue obtained either at biopsy or autopsy.

• Identify the precise type of prion disease (sporadic, familial, or acquired) by examining the prion protein and the prion protein gene, once the diagnosis of prion disease has been established.

• Report findings to caregivers in a timely fashion.

• Transfer the data obtained to the Centers for Disease Control and Prevention (CDC) and the Health Departments of the individual states in order to monitor the prevalence of prion diseases in the USA and investigate possible cases in which the disease has been acquired from other humans or from animals.

• Store tissues for future studies conducted at the NPDPSC as well as at other laboratories around the world.

Diagnostic Activities of the Center:

• In CSF: Search for the presence of the 14-3-3 protein. The 14-3-3 protein is a marker for some prion diseases, such as Creutzfeldt–Jakob disease (CJD), when a number of other neurodegenerative conditions are excluded.

• In DNA extracted from blood, brain, or other tissues: Search for the presence of mutation in the prion protein gene and determine the polymorphism at codon 129 and at other codons.

• In unfixed brain tissue obtained either at biopsy or autopsy: Search for the presence and establish the type of the abnormal, protease-resistant form of the prion protein, also known as scrapie prion protein (PrPSc).

• On fixed brain tissue: Exclude or confirm and characterize the prion disease by microscopic examination following ordinary histological procedures and immunohistochemical demonstration of the prion protein.

Contact information:

• Telephone: (216) 368-0587
• Fax: (216) 368-4090 or (216) 368-2546
• E-mail: cjdsurv@cwru.edu
• Website: http://www.cjdsurveillance.com
• Mail address: National Prion Disease Pathology Surveillance Center, Case Western Reserve University, 2085 Adelbert Road, Room 419, Cleveland, Ohio 44106, USA

Index